Cancer Research in the People's Republic of China and the United States of America

中美两国的癌症研究：

流行病学、病因和治疗新途径

保罗·马克斯医学教授

Grune & Stratton Rapid Manuscript Reproduction

Cancer Research in the People's Republic of China and the United States of America

Epidemiology, Causation and New Approaches to Therapy

Edited by

Paul A. Marks, M.D.

President, Memorial Sloan-Kettering Cancer Center
New York, New York

Formerly, Frode Jensen Professor
Director, Cancer Center/Institute of Cancer Research
Vice President for Health Sciences
Columbia University College of Physicians and Surgeons
New York, New York

Grune & Stratton
A Subsidiary of Harcourt Brace Jovanovich, Publishers
New York   London   Toronto   Sydney   San Francisco

Proceedings of the
Conference on
Cancer Research in the People's Republic of China
and the United States of America
March 28 – 29, 1980

Grune & Stratton, Inc.
111 Fifth Avenue
New York, New York 10003

Distributed in the United Kingdom by
Academic Press Inc. (London) Ltd.
24/48 Oval Road, London NW 1

Library of Congress Catalog Number 80-85070
International Standard Book Number 0-8089-1363-8
Printed in the United States of America

Contents

Cancer Therapy

Acknowledgments

The Conference was supported, in part, by generous gifts from the Armand Hammer Foundation, Pfizer International and the United States – China Lecture Exchange Program of the Committee on Scholarly Communication with the People's Republic of China of the United States National Academy of Sciences and the Scientific and Technical Association of the People's Republic of China.

Many people were involved in the planning for this Conference. It is appropriate to express appreciation to the members of the Program Committee, which included Dr. Xu Bin, Visiting Scientist from the Institute of Materia Medica of the Chinese Academy of Sciences, Shanghai, and Professor I. Bernard Weinstein, University Professor Sol Spiegelman and Professor Emeritus Konrad Hsu of Columbia University. Steven Chen, Joyce Stichman and James Quirk of Columbia University, Robert Feeney and Dr. Greg Gardiner of Pfizer and Philip Wallach associated with Dr. Armand Hammer were all extremely helpful in facilitating the complex arrangements for this Conference.

We are grateful for the cooperation and support received from the Permanent Mission of the People's Republic of China to the United Nations, the Chinese Academy of Medical Sciences and the Chinese Academy of Sciences, as well as our own Department of State, National Cancer Institute and National Academy of Sciences.

Helene Friedman and Mary Corrigan provided their expertise in the editing and preparation of the manuscripts. The staff of Grune & Stratton expedited our publication efforts.

Preface

The first bilateral Conference on Cancer Research in the Peoples Republic of China and the United States was held at Columbia University on the fifth anniversary of the opening of the University's Comprehensive Cancer Center and the Julius and Armand Hammer Health Sciences Center. This volume is composed of those papers delivered by scientists who participated in this conference. In addition, the text includes an address by Dr. Philip Handler, the President of the United States National Academy of Sciences, that was delivered to the participating scientists at a banquet held in their honor.

The aim of the Conference was to provide an opportunity both for individual scientists from the People's Republic of China and the United States to make in-depth presentations of their work and for all participating scientists to explore aspects of particular interest through informal discussion groups.

Those in attendance felt that the Conference made an important contribution to the growing scientific exchange among workers in the area of cancer research in these two countries and to the substantive scientific collaborations that are beginning among individual scientists sharing mutual interests. In fact, four of the participants from the People's Republic of China stayed on in laboratories at the National Cancer Institute, Yale University and Columbia University for collaborative research with members of the faculties of these institutions.

The Conference occurred at a time when advances in the study of cancer epidemiology, biology and therapy in the laboratories of both nations are offering new options for the prevention as well as the treatment of cancer. The timely and useful substantive exchanges among scientists working in these areas of cancer research in our two countries have enabled us to provide detailed reports of data, in several instances previously unpublished, that can be utilized by our colleagues around the world, who are working to decrease the burden of cancer in our society.

Paul A. Marks

Contributors

James Bausch, M.D.
Institute of Cancer Research
College of Physicians and Surgeons
Columbia University
New York, New York

Ronald Berenson
Department of Medicine
University of Utah School of Medicine
Salt Lake City, Utah

Joseph R. Bertino
American Cancer Society Professor of Medicine and Pharmacology
Yale University Medical School
New Haven, Connecticut

William J. Blot
Head of Analytical Studies
Environmental Epidemiology Branch
National Cancer Institute
National Institutes of Health
Bethesda, Maryland

Chang Zhangui
Institute of Materia Medica
Chinese Academy of Medical Sciences
Beijing, China

Bruce Dolnick
Departments of Medicine and Pharmacology
Yale University School of Medicine
New Haven, Connecticut

Renato Dulbecco
The Salk Institute
La Jolla, California

Cecilia Fenoglio
Department of Pathology
College of Physicians and Surgeons
Columbia University
New York, New York

Joseph F. Fraumeni, Jr.
Environmental Epidemiology Branch
National Cancer Institute
National Institutes of Health
Bethesda, Maryland

Han Jui
Institute of Materia Medica
Chinese Academy of Medical Sciences
Beijing, China

Philip Handler
President
National Academy of Sciences
Washington, D.C.

Gertrude Henle
Joseph Stokes, Jr., Research Institute of The Children's Hospital of Philadelphia and
University of Pennsylvania
School of Medicine
Philadelphia, Pennsylvania

Werner Henle
Director, Division of Virology
Joseph Stokes, Jr., Research Institute of The Children's Hospital of Philadelphia
Philadelphia, Pennsylvania

Ji Xiujuan
Institute of Materia Medica
Chinese Academy of Medical Sciences
Beijing, China

Barton A. Kamen
Children's Hospital
Milwaukee, Wisconsin

Yafa Keydar
Faculty of Life Sciences
Department of Microbiology
Tel Aviv University
Ramat Aviv, Israel

Lee Kun
Institute of Materia Medica
Chinese Academy of Medical Sciences
Beijing, China

Li Chen Ch'uan
Associate Professor
Chungshan Medical College
Guangzhou, People's Republic of China

Lin Jun Yao
Institute of Cancer Research
Chinese Academy of Medical Sciences
Beijing, People's Republic of China

Li Min-Hsin
Institute of Cancer Research
Chinese Academy of Medical Sciences
Beijing, People's Republic of China

Li Ping
Institute of Cancer Research
Chinese Academy of Medical Sciences
Beijing, People's Republic of China

Li Zhanrong
Institute of Materia Medica
Chinese Academy of Medical Sciences
Beijing, China

Ricardo Mesa-Tejada
Institute of Cancer Research and
Department of Pathology
College of Physicians and Surgeons
Columbia University
New York, New York

Robert W. Miller
Chief, Clinical Epidemiology Branch
National Cancer Institute
National Institutes of Health
Bethesda, Maryland

Rabindranath Nayak
Institute of Cancer Research
College of Physicians and Surgeons
Columbia University
New York, New York

Tsuneya Ohno
Institute of Cancer Research
College of Physicians and Surgeons
Columbia University
New York, New York

Pan Zhenkun
Institute of Cancer Research
Chinese Academy of Medical Sciences
Beijing, People's Republic of China

Madhava Ramanarayanan
Institute of Cancer Research
College of Physicians and Surgeons
Columbia University
New York, New York

David I. Scheer
Department of Biology
Yale University
New Haven, Connecticut

Sol Spiegelman
Deputy Director for Basic Sciences
Institute of Cancer Research
New York, New York

Sze Chiangyi
Institute of Materia Medica
Chinese Academy of Medical Sciences
Beijing, China

Arthur C. Upton
Department of Environmental Medicine
New York University Medical Center
New York, New York

Wang Yongchao
Institute of Materia Medica
Chinese Academy of Medical Sciences
Beijing, China

I. Bernard Weinstein
Division of Environmental Sciences
Cancer Center/Institute of Cancer Research
Columbia University
College of Physicians and Surgeons
New York, New York

Xu Bin
Institute of Materia Medica
Chinese Academy of Medical Sciences
Shanghai, People's Republic of China

Xu Yuting
Institute of Materia Medica
Chinese Academy of Medical Sciences
Beijing, China

Yao Zhen
Institute of Cell Biology
Chinese Academy of Medical Sciences
Shanghai, People's Republic of China

Zhang Yu Hui
Institute of Cancer Research
Chinese Academy of Medical Sciences
Beijing, People's Republic of China

OPPORTUNITIES AND CHALLENGES
FOR COOPERATION BETWEEN
THE UNITED STATES AND CHINA
IN CANCER RESEARCH

DR. PHILIP HANDLER
President
National Academy of Sciences

ADDRESS*

Thank you very much, Paul, Mr."Hard Guy," Mr. "Easy Guy,"
Mr. Krim, Dr. Hammer, Mr. Ambassador,** distinguished guests,
students all. I am, of course, most pleased to have this
opportunity to be with you this evening to take note of this
unique Conference and to join in celebrating the fifth
anniversary of the Julius and Armand Hammer Center. Particularly, do I wish to congratulate you on this, the first formal
Conference on Cancer Research in China and the U.S. As such,
it constitutes a landmark in the continuing efforts of
scientists in both countries to establish a firm basis for
dialogue and for enduring cooperation and, at the same time,
it underscores the power of science as a medium for bringing
our peoples together. By assembling such a distinguished
group of people to discuss the problems of cancer etiology,
biology, epidemiology, prevention and therapy, Paul Marks has
done us all a great service.

---

*   This address was delivered at the Banquet honoring the
scientists from the People's Republic of China and the United
States on Cancer Research in the Rotunda of Low Library,
Columbia University, March 28, 1980. Dr. Philip Handler was
introduced by Dr. Paul Marks, Vice President for Health
Sciences and Director of the Cancer Center, Columbia University.

**   Mr. Arthur Krim, Chairman of the Board of Trustees,
Columbia University; Dr. Armand Hammer, President of the
Armand Hammer Foundation; Mr. Ambassador, Lai Ya-Li, Permanent
Mission of the People's Republic of China to the United
Nations.

1

Research on cancer is a high national priority in the United States as, I understand, it is in China also. By combining our understanding, in meetings such as this, and by continuing the exchange of scientists and scientific information between our two countries, we will, I hope, advance the worldwide search for the causes and cures for cancer.

In the eight years since the signing of the Shanghai Communique, our two countries have come a long way in establishing a viable political and economic relationship. Relations in scientific and technical fields have evolved from the "scientific tourism" of the period 1972 to about 1977, to more rewarding forms of exchange—such as this conference. We have moved from a pattern of brief, survey visits by delegations to exchange of individual research scholars and lecturers for meaningful periods and the convening of substantive bilateral scientific symposia such as this and the recent symposium on polymer chemistry in Peking. Much will be gained, I am sure, from the continuing exchange of ideas and scientific data and from the longer-term visits of scholars for specific research projects.

A few weeks ago, in Peking, as a member of the binational commission on science and technology, I signed an agreement with the Chinese Academy of Sciences on behalf of the National Academy of Sciences including the National Academy of Engineering and the Institute of Medicine. This "Memorandum of Understanding," signed only one year after the normalization of diplomatic relations between the United States and China, calls for mutually beneficial programs of scholarly cooperation. Joint programs sponsored by our two academies of science will take such forms as exchanges of individual scholars, bilateral seminars and symposia, discussions of long-range planning, and exchange of publications. We shall also serve as mechanisms for facilitating the personal plans of independent investigators as we already serve as a coordinating mechanism with respect to the placement of students and postdocs.

As you may know, the National Academy of Sciences has had a Committee on Scholarly Communication with the People's Republic of China since 1966. Since 1972 this Committee has sponsored exchanges in many fields of basic and applied science, the social sciences, and the humanities. Medical exchanges, particularly in cancer research, were no small part of that program. In fact, one of the first breaks away from "scholarly tourism" was the 1977 visit to China of the Committee's Cancer Delegation, led by Dr. Henry Kaplan of Stanford University. I am happy to note that several members of that group are in the room tonight (Dr. Bertino, Dr. Miller, Dr. Weinstein). Their presence here attests to their continuing interest in opportunities for cancer research in China.

Dr. Kaplan's delegation proposed four areas of potential opportunities for cooperation in cancer research, four areas that offer great challenge to the scientists of both countries.

First was EPIDEMIOLOGY.

We have the good fortune to have with us tonight Dr. Li Bing, Vice Director of the Institute for Cancer Research, Chinese Academy of Medical Sciences, Peking. Dr. Li is here under the auspices of the Lecture Exchange Program of the Academy's China Committee.

Dr. Li's research on geographic patterns of cancer in China, especially her work on esophageal cancer in north China, is known throughout the world. Her presentation this morning on regional patterns of cancer as clues to causation and prevention offer hope that such investigations in China will lead to new etiological discoveries which may have implications for people throughout the world. We have much to learn from the observational techniques of Chinese scientists, and a promising beginning could be made in collaborative studies on the regional cancer patterns in China and in the United States.

Second was CARCINOGENESIS.

Guided by epidemiological investigations, studies into possible carcinogenic substances in the regional high-risk cancer areas are potential subjects for collaborative ventures. Dr. Li Ming Xin (Shin) has reported on the possible role of nitrosamines and their precursors in the drinking water and foodstuffs of the inhabitants of the high-risk area for esophageal cancer. Further investigations on this topic and on other possible environmental carcinogens--in China and in the United States--might provide insights that will illuminate the etiology of cancer. And we badly need such. I say that because I am persuaded that some profound simplifying concept has been eluding us. Let me explain why.

The general question is: Need there be an external
etiological agent to initiate carcinogenesis, or is the
neoplastic process frequently the mere consequence of having
lived long enough to permit the appearance of cancer as an
expression of events necessitated by our own biology? What
are the paramount relevant facts?

First, the median age of death due to cancer, worldwide,
is much the same, just over 69 years, and has not been changing in any significant way. If due to exposure to some agent,
decades before, what happens during that long hiatus? What
biological clock governs these events?

Second, as a fraction of all deaths, death due to cancer
has been rising everywhere in the world in which industrialization and sanitation are taking hold. As infectious
diseases, nutritional diseases, endocrine diseases, etc., are
brought under control, and the life expectancy of the population rises, deaths due to cancer come to loom larger and
larger as a fraction of the total. But the age-corrected
incidence of cancer has not shown dramatic changes. In the
United States, it actually fell significantly from 1950 to
1971 but has been rising slowly since then.

Third, a series of circumstances combined to direct our
attention to environmental factors. Primary among these was
the highly disparate site-specific distribution of different
forms of cancer around the world and, indeed, within regions
in the same country. On the well-founded assumption that
there do not appear to be any strong genetic predispositions
to one or another form of cancer associated with specific
ethnic or racial groups, these differences in site-specific
cancer distribution strongly suggested the operation of
"environmental factors" in perhaps three-quarters of all
cancer. But what are these "environmental factors"? Diverse
studies conducted in laboratories around the world have
focused attention on specific chemical carcinogens and
mutagens. Awareness of the steadily increasing dissemination
of thousands of man-made chemicals and of the pollutants
associated with modern industry led some to propose that
these are major contributors to environmental carcinogenesis.
In fact, however, no evidence supports that thesis, except in
those relatively rare instances where a specific form of
cancer occurs with a high incidence among individuals subject
to unusually high occupational exposure to some noxious
chemical such as vinyl chloride, for example.

There are certainly contrary arguments that give one
pause. The seeming causal association of cancer occurrence
with the industrialization process is denied by the fact that
the age-corrected incidence of cancer, around the world, in

countries for which such data are reasonably reliable, shows
absolutely no correlation with income per capita or with
energy use per capita, simple indicators of the extent of
industrialization and, hence, of potential exposure to diverse
chemicals. Rather, the gross incidence of cancer rises simply
as life expectancy rises.

One can come at the question another way. In order to
appreciate whether, indeed, most carcinogenesis may be the
consequence of chemical insult, one would like to be able to
relate cancer incidence or cancer mortality to the dose-
response relationships for known carcinogens. At this time
just over 20% of all Americans die of cancer. The question,
therefore, becomes what dose of chemical carcinogen is
required to produce such a result. Unfortunately, the dose-
response curves for most known chemical carcinogens have been
studied so inadequately that it is not possible to state that
relationship with any confidence. But there is one carcinogen
for which such data are known rather well, i.e., that for
ionizing radiation. Data are available from large numbers of
test animals and, regrettably, also available for the survivors of the bombs dropped at Hiroshima and Nagasaki. For the
latter we can state the answer to our question rather pre-
cisely. The single radiation dose required is close to the
LD_{50}; that is to say, after a single acute dose, such that
approximately half of the exposed individuals would die of
acute radiation disease within a few weeks, an additional
one-fifth of the survivors will ultimately die of cancer.
If one asks what chronic exposure is required to obtain the
same end point, then animal data indicate that the answer is
approximately 100-200 times background radiation daily throughout the life of the exposed individual. This is sufficient
radiation to induce one or two defects in the structure of the
DNA of every cell in the body, every day of the animal's life.
Yet, in the end, only one-fifth of such animals will die of
cancer. Patently, the overwhelming bulk of those defects are
either repaired or silent, i.e. find no observable expression.
I cannot know whether the kinds of defects created by ionizing
radiation bear any relationship to the actual mechanism of any
chemical carcinogen. If there be any analogy, it will be
apparent that the dose required to achieve the actual known
end point in man, 20% mortality, must be rather large. But if
that is the case, why have we failed to identify the responsible carcinogens anywhere in the human environment? There
are, indeed, naturally occurring carcinogens--"initiators" in
current parlance. And there are "promoters", but in amounts
so small that one finds it extremely difficult to relate these
to the incidence of cancer among our population. None of

which is to gainsay the possibility of quite specific environmental causes operative in quite specific circumstances as,
for example, the possibility of a real chemical carcinogen
responsible for the high rate of esophageal cancer in north
China or in certain regions of Iran.

I note these contradictions not to confuse you but to
suggest that there is something about the etiology of cancer
which we have simply failed to grasp. And I join with John
Higginson of the International Cancer Agency in Lyons, France,
in believing that no more than 5 to 10% of all cancer can,
indeed, be the consequence of the sum of the influences of
genuine chemical carcinogens--present in the natural environment or man-made--together with radiation--natural and man-
made. Although "environmental factors" surely bear somehow
on much of the rest of cancer, these factors must be assumed
to reside in sometimes subtle, sometimes gross aspects of
"lifestyle"; for example, the extent to which one smokes,
drinks alcohol, imbibes coffee or tea, or unsaturated fat or
total fat, or fiber, or some particular unusual foodstuff
which need contain no material that would seem to be an
initiator. Surely relevant are sexual habits, the age at
which sex is initiated and the age at which babies are born,
with their resultant effects on hormonal balances. But with
the exception, perhaps, of smoking, this suggests that much
of carcinogenesis occurs without requirement for an external
primary initiator. And if that be true, it is time to return
to the search for the natural mechanism which is at play.
And that is a huge challenge for the scientists of all
countries--ours included.

The third area proposed for cooperation was NEW DRUG
DEVELOPMENT.

China possesses a wealth of plants that have been
employed in traditional Chinese medicine. Research intended
to identify the active ingredients of these natural products
is now under way in China, I understand. In the past several
years, the Academy's China Committee has sponsored several
exchanges focusing on new drug development, especially new
drugs from natural products. Combining the resources and the
technology of both countries in the search for new drugs,
including, hopefully, new anti-tumor drugs from plants,
should be a high priority.

Fourth, BASIC BIOLOGICAL RESEARCH.

In the search for understanding of cancer, there is much
to be done in basic studies in cell biology, immunology,
virology, molecular biology, biochemistry, genetics and
related fields. Years of research await us. I have read of
some excellent biological research in Chinese institutes,

and am aware of the eagerness of many Chinese scientists to upgrade their own competence and the capabilities of their laboratories and then get on with such science. I am sure that I speak for all my colleagues here tonight when I say that we welcome the opportunity for collaboration between American and Chinese scientists in this important field.

Finally, let me reiterate my belief in the profound importance of international scientific communication. For many years, Americans were out of touch with scientists in China; we are just beginning to make up for lost time. I am proud of the record of the National Academy of Sciences' exchanges with China, including in areas relating to cancer research. I have noted several areas of cancer research which offer signal opportunities for future collaboration between scientists in China and the United States as part of the worldwide effort. These opportunities constitute a challenge which will only be met by steady determination. The ultimate goal is to reduce the ravages of a disease that afflicts not only the peoples of our two countries, but all mankind. At the same time, this joint effort should help forge human bridges of understanding that will cross the barriers of cultural and political difference, and, in some small measure, contribute therefore to the universal cause of world peace.

Thank you.

Cancer Epidemiology: Causation

OVERVIEW: CANCER RESEARCH*

PAUL A. MARKS, M.D.
Frode Jensen Professor
Director,
Cancer Center/Institute of Cancer Research
Vice President for Health Sciences
Columbia University
College of Physicians and Surgeons
New York City 10032

*Studies referred to in this manuscript performed in the laboratory of the author, were supported in part by grants from the United States National Cancer Institute (CA-13696 and CA-18314) and the American Cancer Society (Ch-68A).

In the People's Republic of China and in the United States cancer is the third and the second most common causes of death for the population as a whole, respectively. In both China and in the United States there is an increased appreciation that environmental factors may play a role in the cause of the most common kinds of cancers (1-5).

EPIDEMIOLOGY OF CANCER

One of the most striking aspects of the cancer problem is the variation in incidence of different forms of cancers in different geograhic areas. In the United States roughly half of all cancer deaths are caused by cancers of three organs: lung, large intestine and breast (4,5). In China the most common causes of death from cancer are stomach, esophagus and liver (3). In some geographic areas of China, cancers which are among the rarer types in this country, are quite common, as for example, nasalpharyngeal carcinoma (6).

Evidence that suggest that environmental factors play an important role in the cause of cancer is derived, in part, from epidemiological studies of the distribution of different types of cancer. Among the most interesting epidemiological studies in this regard are those which have been pursued in China for the past several years and are providing a detailed analysis of the distribution, by incidence and type, of cancers for a large population group (3).

STUDIES ON MIGRANT POPULATIONS

Other epidemiological evidence with respect to the possible contribution of environmental factors to the cause of cancer derives from several types of studies. Among such studies are analysis of the incidence of different forms of cancer among populations and their offspring which migrate from one country to another. In these studies, some idea can be obtained as to the genetic and nongenetic factors, and, to some extent, the time course of induction of cancer. For example, death rates from cancer of the stomach, liver, colon and prostate among male Japanese immigrants to California and these immigrants' sons born in California tend consistently toward California norms (Table 1) (7). It appears to require more than one generation for the profiles for age-adjusted death rates from these cancers among the Japanese populations to be similar to geographically contiguous California whites. Since intermarriage among the immigrant Japanese population is high, these data suggest environmental rather than genetic factors, play a major role in accounting for the changes in incidence.

TABLE 1

Age-adjusted death rates for various cancers observed among male Japanese in Japan, male Japanese immigrants to California and these immigrants' sons born in California. The results are expressed as the ratio of the number of deaths that occurred, divided by the number that would have been expected in a similar group of California whites.

Cancer Site	Death rates among Japanese (ratio to death rates in California Whites)		
	Japan	Immigrants to California	Sons of Immigrants
Stomach	6.5	4.6	3.0
Liver	3.7	2.1	2.2
Colon	0.2	0.8	0.9
Prostrate	0.1	0.5	1.0

Adapted from (5) p. 50. Source (7).

Similar conclusions are suggested by studies of Jewish populations who migrated to Israel from Europe or from the United States. Among these populations the immigrants tend to maintain the incidence of different types of cancer that is typical of their country of birth, while their Israeli born children have a much lower incidence of almost all kinds of cancer (Table 2) (8). In this regard the immigrant children become more like the indigenous Israeli population and Jewish immigrants from Asia and Africa among whom the overall incidence of cancer is somewhat lower than in the United States.

TABLE 2

Overall age-adjusted incidence for all forms of cancer among four groups in Israel, 1961-65, compared to the incidence in the United States.

Group	Population	Incidence per 100,000 Males	Females
non-Jews (mostly Arabs)	140,000	179	93
Jews born in Israel	425,000	193	195
Jews born in Africa or elsewhere in Asia	291,000	208	167
Jews born in the U.S. or Europe	352,000	294	313
General U.S. population		300-400	300-400

Adapted from (5) p. 51. Source (8).

CANCER AND AGING

Cancer has a higher incidence among older people. For example, the death rates from cancer in the United States increased more than a hundred fold between the ages of 25 and 80 (9). Various models have been proposed for the clustering of cancer in older people (10,11). One reasonable theory of carcinogenesis suggests that it involves a multi-step process and cancer will not occur until each of these steps such as mutation of several genes has occurred. This theory predicts that the log of cancer incidence should be linearly related to the log of age. This relationship of incidence to age is in fact observed for deaths from malignant neoplasms, such as in the United States between ages 25 and 80 (Figure 1) (5,9,10).

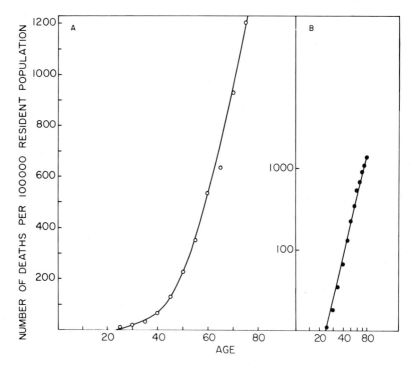

Figure 1:   *Death rates due to malignant neoplasms,*
                United States, 1977. a) linear scale;
                b) logarithmic scale (9).

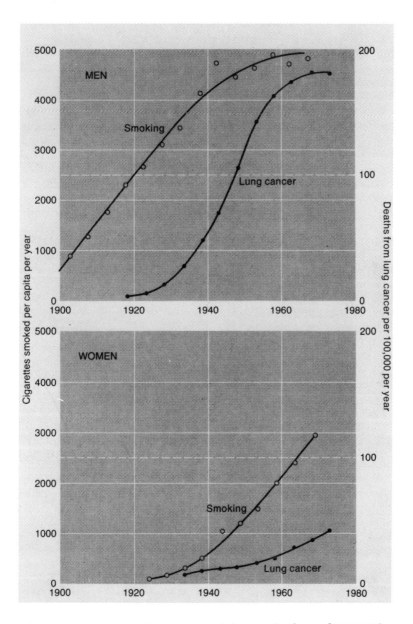

Figure 2:   Relation between smoking and the subsequent
              rise in the death rate from lung cancer for
              men and women in England (from (5) p. 45).

TIME COURSE OF DEVELOPMENT OF CANCERS

There is a considerable amount of data to indicate that
a lag period of many years may occur between exposure to a
potential carcinogen and the appearance of a tumor. This lag
has been suggested for a number of carcinogens including
ionizing and those related to smoking (Figure 2) (12,13).
This lag may be 5 to 30 years or more between exposure and
the appearance of cancer and has several import implications
for the mechanism of carcinogenesis. It is consistent with
the hypothesis that a given cancer may have several factors
contributing to its cause (14). Knowledge of the relationship
between age and death from cancer does not tell us what causes
a cancer, it only suggests that there may be two or more
events in the course of development of clinically evident
cancer over a period of years.

It is attractive to speculate that these accumulated
events, represent changes at the level of DNA structure,
transmitted through a cell lineage. In theory, environmental
factors could cause changes in DNA which alter normal control
of cell replication and expression of differentiated characteristics. Alternatively, a genetically determined factor(s)
could increase susceptibility of cells to transformation to
abnormal growth. Transmission of a "susceptibility" to
cancer through the germ cell line is, of course, not incom-
patible with environmental factors playing a role in the
transformation of cells to cancer cells.

GENETIC FACTORS AND CANCER

There is evidence that genetic determinants may play
a role in oncogenesis. For example, there are individuals
who have a greatly increased risk for some kinds of cancers,
such as the gene for polyposis of the colon which markedly
increases the age related incidence of cancer of the colon
(15). One hundred percent of persons with this gene get colon
cancer by age 40, while only 3% of the general population
get this disease by age 100 (Figure 3). Other examples are
the inherited defect in the enzymes that repair DNA damaged
by ultraviolet light, the xeroderma pigmentosum, syndromes
which are associated with a high incidence of multiple skin
cancers. There are several genetically determined defects
in DNA replication or repair which appear to lead to an increased susceptibility incidence to various types of cancers
(16). Our understanding has not yet proceeded to the point
where we can identify the specific enzyme defect in any of
these syndromes.

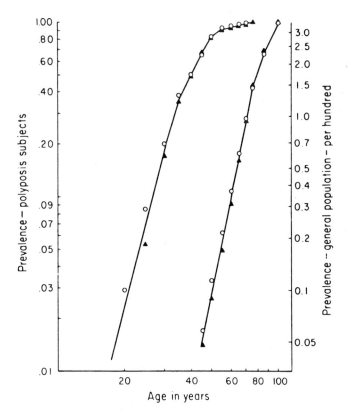

Figure 3:   Carcinoma of the colon. A comparison of the
age-specific prevalences among polyposis coli
subjects (left) and all subjects (right).
(▲) Male; (o) Female (11).

Studies on the metabolism of various drugs employing comparisons between monozygotic and dizygotic twins suggest that genetic factors are important determinants in the metabolism of various drugs and by extrapolation, probably carcinogenic agents as well (17). These studies do not define the specific genetically controlled trait affecting metabolism of one or another substance. These studies do raise a number of questions with respect to the potential efficacy of screening programs to identify individuals with increased susceptibility to various environmental hazards. Our science base in these areas is inadequate to provide a sound approach to the problem of individual risk assessment with respect to susceptibility to cancer in relation to exposure to different environmental hazards.

VIRUSES AND CANCER

The concept that viruses may be involved in carcinogenesis is based on a number of observations including the fact that certain leukemia-like diseases of lower animal forms including chickens, cats and inbred strains of mice and rats can be induced by innoculating them with viruses isolated from leukemic animals. At the present time, there is no unambiguous evidence that any class of human cancers is regularly caused by a virus. Some cancers are often associated with elevated levels of antibody to certain viruses (6,18,19). Some cancer cells have been shown to contain viral nucleic acid sequences. Certain cancers occasionally arise in clusters of cases which some investigators have suggested could reflect an infectious (e.g. viral) factor in their etiology.

THERAPY

Epidemiological and genetic studies bear on questions of causes of cancer and on prospects for prevention of cancers. The cancer problem is also being approached by investigations on the nature of the mechanisms of transformation of cells and prospects for developing more effective approaches to the therapy of cancer. Studies on the mechanism of carcinogenesis (20-24) and experimental cancer therapy (25-28) are presented in detail in several papers in this volume.

At the present time there is no effective general cure for cancer and no sign that one is about to be discovered. Several cancers can, under certain circumstances, be apparently cured by a combination of therapeutic approaches including the use of cytotoxic drugs. Certain new approaches to therapy may be suggested from the investigations of our Chinese colleagues over the past several years on the identification, isolation and therapeutic experience with agents derived, in part, from traditional Chinese herbs that have been used in the treatment of neoplastic diseases (26,28).

MECHANISM OF CARCINOGENESIS

The nature of the process of carcinogenesis is an area of intensive investigation. Cancer cells appear in certain instances, to have a defect in the mechanisms that control the expression of genes for differentiation characteristics and control of cell growth. Our own laboratory (29,30) has been concerned with the control of gene expression in transformed cells using as our particular model for study, the Friend virus transformed mouse erythroleukemia cell system. In addition to investigating the nature of the block to normal erythroid differentiation associated with the virus infection of these mouse cells, research on this system has led to the identification of a number of low molecular weight chemicals, such as hexamethylene bisacetamide, which can induce these cells to express differentiated characteristics and lose their oncogenic properties. This is an area of research which is of interest in that it may provide clues to an approach to the treatment of cancer employing agents that are not cytotoxic, but rather induce patterns of cell differentiation similar to that of normal cell lines.

CANCER DETECTION

Another aspect of the cancer problem dealt with in this volume (6,18,19) concerns a most important question for the cancer patient, namely whether cancer can be systematically detected at a sufficiently early stage to permit curative therapy. Efforts are being made in the United States and in the People's Republic of China, to develop screening programs that will detect specific cancers at an early stage in development. With certain types of cancer these programs are having limited, but significant, success. In the realm of preventive medicine, issues related to screening become of critical importance. We must understand the applicability as well as the limitations of these programs.

CONCLUSION

The cancer problem arouses much interest. All too often expectations have been raised which have not been realized with respect to advances in prevention, in diagnosis or in treatment. There are no shortcuts to progress in this area.

All of us involved in research in this area have a heavy responsibility to be aware of the best understanding of the nature of the cancer problem and the opportunities for approaching solutions to the questions. Open scientific exchange such as occurred at the Conference which lead to the publication of this volume is an important part of the process of developing new opportunities to advance our understanding of cancer prevention, diagnosis and treatment.

REFERENCES

1. Doll, R. *Prevention of Cancer, Pointers from Epidemiology.* The Muffield Provincial Hospital Trust, London (1967).
2. Fraumeni, J.F., Jr. *Epidemiological Studies of Cancer Carcinogens: Identification and Mechanisms of Action.* (ed. A. Clark Griffin and Charles R. Shaw). Raven Press, New York, pp. 51-63 (1979).
3. Li Ping. *This volume.*
4. Heatt, H.H., Watson, T.D., and Winsten, J.A. *Origins of Human Cancer.* Cold Spring Harbor Conferences on Cell Proliferation. *Vol. 4,* (1977).
5. Cairns, J. *Cancer: Science and Society.* W.H. Freeman and Company, San Francisco (1978).
6. Li Chen-Ch'uan. *This volume.*
7. Buell, P. and Dunn, J.E. *Cancer 18:* 656-664 (1965).
8. Doll, R., Muir, C. and Waterhouse, J. *Cancer Incidence in Five Continents.* UICC Springer-Verlag, Berlin (1970).
9. *Health: United States 1979,* U.S. Department of Health, Education and Welfare. DHEW Publication No. (DHS)80-1232 pp. 105.
10. Armitage, P. and Doll, R. *Stochastic Models for Carcinogenis.* Proc. Fourth Berkeley Symposium on Mathematical Statistics and Probability. *4:* 19-38, Berkeley and Los Angeles, University of California Press (1961).
11. Knudson, A.G., Jr. Genetic and Environmental Interactions in the Origin of Human Cancer *in Progress in Cancer Research and Therapy 3:* 391-400 (1977).
12. Doll, R. *Cancer Res. 38:* 3573-3583 (1978).
13. Jablon, S. and Kato, H. *Radiation Res. 50:* 649-698(1972).
14. Hegginsar, J. *J. Natl. Cancer Institute 63:* 1291-1298 (1979).
15. Ashley, D.J.B. *J. Med. Genet. 3:* 376-378 (1969).
16. Cleaver, J.E. Human Diseases with In Vitro Manifestations of Altered Repair and Replication of DNA *in Progress in Cancer Research and Therapy 3:* 355-364 (1977).

17. Vesell, E.S. Twin Studies in Pharmacogenetics, *Human Genetics Supplement 1:* 19-30 (1978).
18. Spiegelman, S. *This volume.*
19. Henle, W. *This volume.*
20. Dulbecco, R. *This volume.*
21. Yao Zhen. *This volume.*
22. Li Mingxin. *This volume.*
23. Weinstein, I.B. *This volume.*
24. Axel, R. *This volume.*
25. Osserman, E.F. *This volume.*
26. Xu Bin. *This volume.*
27. Bertino, J. *This volume.*
28. Han Jui. *This volume.*
29. Marks, P.A. and Rifkind, R.A. Erythroleukemic Differentiation. *Annual Rev. of Biochem. 47:* 419-448 (1978).
30. Rifkind, R.A., Fibach, E., Maniatis, G., Gambari, R. and Marks. Commitment to differentiation of normal and transformed erythroid precursors *in Cellular and Molecular Regulation of Hemoglobin Switching* (ed. G. Stamatoyannopoulos and A. Nienhuis) Grune & Stratton, New York, pp. 421-436 (1979).

EVOLVING PERSEPECTIVES ON THE
EPIDEMIOLOGY AND BIOLOGY OF CANCER:
NEEDS AND OPPORTUNITIES

ARTHUR C. UPTON, M.D.
New York University Medical Center
Institute of Environmental Medicine
New York, New York

Thank you, Dr. Marks. It is a pleasure and privilege for me to chair this opening session in the Conference, and to reiterate words of welcome to our Chinese colleagues, many of whom have journeyed long distances to be with us today.

The first session, as you know, deals with cancer epidemiology and biology. As Dr. Marks has brought out, this aspect of cancer research presents us with enormous opportunity as well as challenge.

There are marked differences in the incidence of cancer in different parts of the world (Table 1, Fig. 1). These do not reflect static patterns. The risks do not apply equally to all individuals in a given population. Within any one country, the risks may vary from place to place and from time to time.

As Dr. Marks mentioned, there has been an epidemic of lung cancer in the U.S. within the last 50 years, which has followed an increase in cigarette consumption, first in males and then in females (Fig. 2). Moreover, the relation between the excess in risk and the number of cigarettes smoked per day indicates that there may be no threshold for the carcinogenic effects of cigarette smoking (Fig. 3).

The implications of this dose-effect relationship are far-reaching, since the carcinogens present in cigarette smoke are also encountered from many other sources. Further evidence implying non-threshold dose-effect relationships has come from studies of radiation carcinogenesis in a number of irradiated human populations (U.N., 1977), as I will mention later.

Simultaneous with the increase in the occurrence of lung cancer during the past fifty years, there has been an almost equally dramatic decrease in the incidence of stomach cancer (Fig. 4). The reasons for this decrease are obscure, but many observers postulate that it may have resulted from improved nutrition. In Japan, where the incidence of stomach cancer is still appreciably higher than in the U.S., the

23

TABLE 1

Range of Geographic Variation in the Incidence of Common Cancers[a]

Type of Cancer	High-incidence area	Cumulative risk[b] (%)	Range of variation[c]	Low-incidence area
Skin	Australia, Queensland	>20	>200	India, Bombay
Esophagus	Iran, N.E.	20	300	Nigeria
Bronchus	England	11	35	Nigeria
Stomach	Japan	11	25	Uganda
Cervix uteri	Colombia	10	15	Israel, Jewish
Liver	Mozambique	8	70	Norway
Prostrate	USA, black	7	30	Japan
Breast (female)	USA, Connecticut	7	5	Uganda
Colon	USA, Connecticut	3	10	Nigeria
Buccal cavity	India, part	>2	>25	Denmark
Rectum	Denmark	2	20	Nigeria
Bladder	USA, Connecticut	2	4	Japan
Ovary	Denmark	2	8	Japan
Corpus uteri	USA, Connecticut	2	10	Japan
Nasopharynx	Singapore, Chinese	2	40	England
Pancreas	New Zealand, Maori	2	5	Uganda
Penis	Uganda, part	1	300	Israel, Jewish

a From Doll, 1977.
b By 75 years of age in absence of other causes of death.
c At ages 35-64 years.

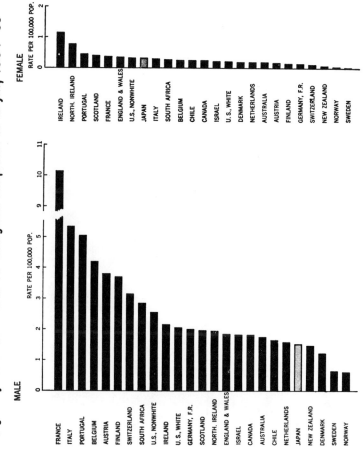

Fig. 1. Age-adjusted death rates for malignant neoplasms of the larynx, 1964 – 1965 (from Segi, 1969).

25

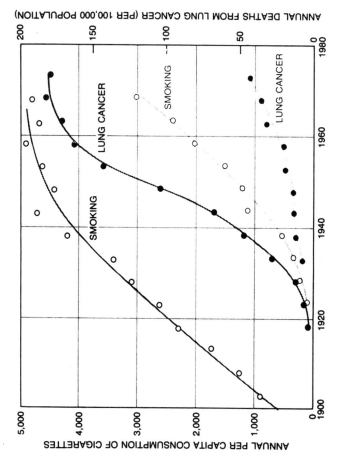

Fig. 2. Time-trends in lung cancer mortality and cigarette consumption, in England and Wales *(from Cairns, 1975).*

26

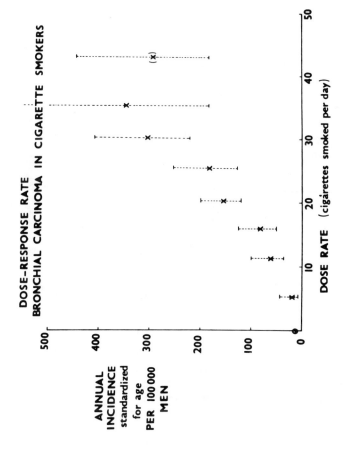

Fig. 3. *Incidence of lung cancer in regular cigarette smokers in relation to the number of cigarettes smoked per day (from Doll, 1978).*

27

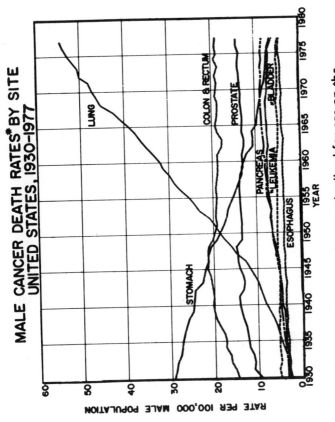

*Rate for the male population standardized for age on the
1940 U.S. population. Sources of Data: National Vital
Statistics Division and Bureau of the Census, United States.

Fig. 4. *Time-trends in cancer death rates in U.S. males,
standardized for age (from Am. Cancer Soc., 1980).*

incidence now appears to be declining; however, there have
been so many changes in the Japanese diet within recent years
that no simple correlation is possible (Fig. 5). Moreover,
as we all know, Japanese youngsters are larger today than
they were 30 years ago, go through menarche at an earlier age,
and, in fact, exhibit various metabolic changes that may be
related to dietary alterations.

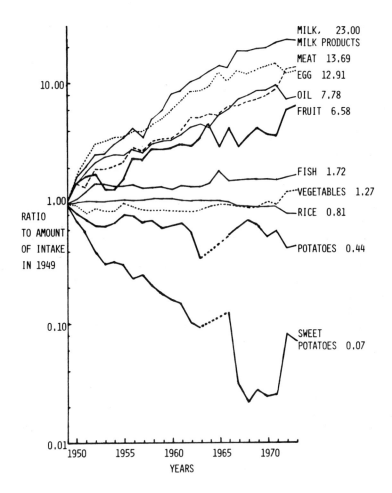

Fig. 5. *Changes in dietary intake of certain foods in Japan,
1949-1973 (from Hirayama, 1977).*

As we consider the role of environmental risk factors, in general, one of the most noteworthy recent developments is the fact that the correlation between mutagenicity and carci-nogenicity has gotten progressively better with improvements in assay technique which provide for appropriate activation of carcinogens (Fig. 6). The mutagenicity of most carcinogens enables powerful new approaches for the detection of cancer-causing substances. Elucidation of carcinogen activation pathways also provides valuable new insights into the basis for differences in susceptibility among individuals, and promising new possibilities for blocking the action of carcinogens as a strategy for cancer prevention.

It is significant that in atomic-bomb survivors of Hiroshima, the incidence of leukemia appears to increase as linear nonthreshold function of the radiation dose, even at the lowest dose levels investigated. Although this would not appear to be true of survivors in Nagasaki, for whom the data point to a curvilinear response (Fig. 7), the difference is explicable on radiobiological grounds in view of the fact that the radiations at Hiroshima included a large neutron component, while those at Nagasaki were composed almost entirely of gamma rays.

Neutrons are more effective in transforming cells in vitro (Fig. 8) than are X-rays or gamma rays. Similarly, the genetic effects of neutrons characteristically increase as a linear function of the dose, whereas they increase linearly with X-rays only in the low dose region. To explain the upward curvature of the X-ray response at intermediate doses (Fig. 9), it is postulated that a single X-ray traversal of the cell nucleus seldom deposits enough energy within a critical volume to cause irreparable damage to DNA, in contrast to a neutron traversal, while two or more X-ray traversals can do so if they are close enough together in space and time.

Since the dose-effect curve for sparsely ionizing radiations bends upward in the intermediate dose region for many types of effects, linear extrapolation from observations at high doses will tend to overestimate the risks of such effects at low doses and low dose rates (Fig. 10). In the case of breast cancer, however, the risk per unit dose is no smaller in women who received repeated fluoroscopic examinations of the chest during treatment for pulmonary tuberculosis than in atomic bomb survivors and women treated with X-ray therapy for acute postpartum mastitis (Fig. 11), despite the fact that the dose to the breast in the fluoroscoped women was only of the order of a few rads per examination, received once every 2-3 weeks, and spread out over a period of months

or years. The occurrence of essentially the same carcinogenic effect to the breast in all groups implies a linear
dose-effect relationship. Hence, the same dose-effect model
may not be applicable to both breast cancer and leukemia.

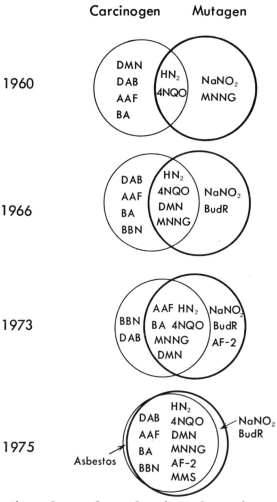

Fig. 6. Chronology of overlapping of carcinogenicity and
mutagenicity (from Sugimura et al, 1976).

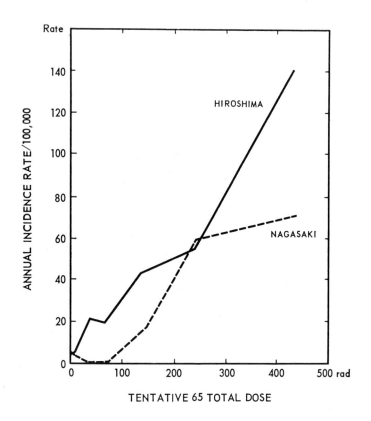

Fig. 7. *Incidence of leukemia in atomic-bomb survivors in relation to radiation dose (from Ishimaru et al, 1971).*

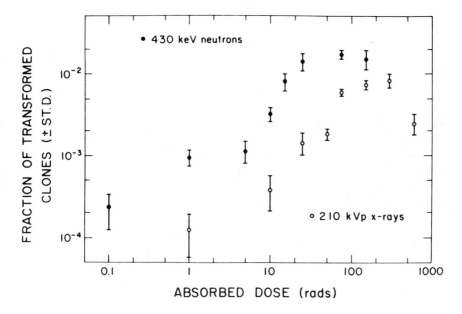

Fig. 8. Frequency of hamster embryo cell transformation in relation to dose of X-rays or fast neutrons (from Borek, 1976).

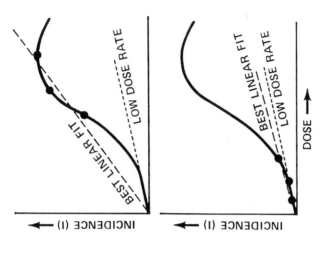

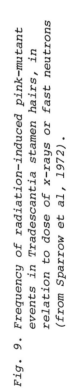

Fig. 10. Schematic illustration of how linear extrapolation from data at high doses and high dose rates can over-estimate risks at low doses if the dose-response relation is actually a linear-quadratic function (from Brown, 1977).

Fig. 9. Frequency of radiation-induced pink-mutant events in Tradescantia stamen hairs, in relation to dose of x-rays or fast neutrons (from Sparrow et al, 1972).

34

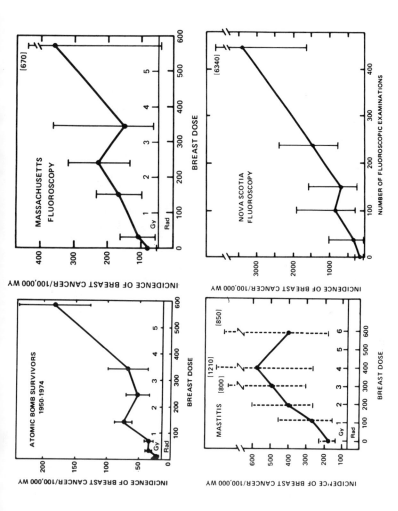

Fig. 11. Dose-incidence curves for breast cancer in relation to radiation exposure, in women surviving atomic-bomb radiation, women treated with X-rays for acute postpartum mastitis, and women subjected to multiple fluoroscopic examinations for pulmonary tuberculosis (from Boice et al, 1979).

35

To account for the observed carcinogenic effects of radiation and to assess the risk of other cancer-causing agents, we obviously need better knowledge of the mechanisms of carcinogenesis. In approaching this problem, we must envision the cancer process to evolve stepwise (Fig. 12), involving initial changes which may be equivalent to mutation-like events but also involving additional changes before the transformational damage becomes fully expressed in affected cells. Moreover, when the dose of any carcinogen is large enough, it may cause such gross damage to tissues as to profoundly alter the cellular environment, change hormone levels, affect immunological responsiveness, and disturb other functions. Hence, the predominant effect of a carcino-gen may vary with the dose. Other modifying factors may also affect the response. As a result of these influences, the shape of the dose-effect curve may be highly complicated. Until we understand the entire process better, it will be extremely difficult for us to arrive at adequate explanations or confident estimates of the risks of carcinogenic effects at low doses.

Despite the gaps in our knowledge, available evidence on the carcinogenic effects of radiation allows us to make tentative estimates of risks in the low dose domain. Accord-ing to such estimates, the risks for different organs vary appreciably, with the female breast appearing to be the most sensitive tissue in the adult (Tables 2,3), for reasons which remain to be disclosed. Twenty years ago, we would not have imagined the breast to be so sensitive, based on the data available at that time. Leukemia was then the cancer of chief concern.

The availability of quantitative estimates (Tables 2,3), even with their severe limitations, is helpful in assessing the potential risks from radiation, as compared with hazards of other types. For example, one can estimate the fraction of cancer in the general population that might be attributable to radiation from medical and dental examinations, nuclear power, and other man-made sources, as compared with natural background radiation (Table 4). Taking all of these sources together, it would appear that exposure of the population to ionizing radiation may account for only about 2-3 percent of the total cancer incidence. Any attempt to detect an effect so small by studying the variations in cancer rates that might be attributable to differences in natural background radiation levels would greatly exceed the capacity of existing epidemiological techniques. We can arrive at such risk estimates only by extrapolation, based on our concepts of dose-effect relationships and mechanisms.

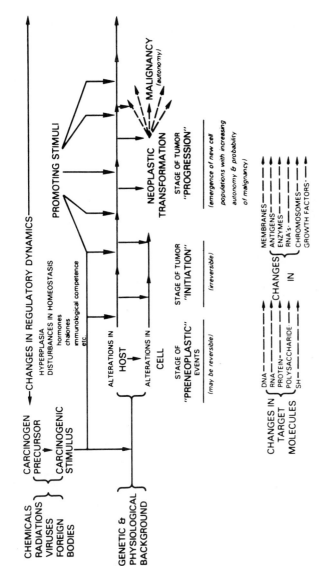

Fig. 12. Schematic representation of the sequence of events envisioned to occur in the development of a cancer (from Upton, 1978).

TABLE 2

Assumed Parameters of Model for Estimating Cancer Risks Associated with
Low-Level Ionizing Radiation (From Nat. Acad. Sci., 1972).

Age at Irradiation	Type of Cancer	Duration of Latent Period (years)	Duration of Plateau Region (years)[a]	Risk Estimate	
				Absolute Risk[b] (deaths/10^6/ yr/rem)	Relative Risk (% increase in deaths/rem)
In Utero	Leukemia	0	10	25	50
	All other cancer	0	10	25	50
0-9 Years	Leukemia	2	25	2.0	5.0
	All other cancer	15	(a)30 (b)Life	1.0	2.0
10 + Years	Leukemia	2	25	1.0	2.0
	All other cancer	15	(a)30 (b)Life	5.0	0.2

a Plateau region = interval following latent period during which risk remains elevated.

b The absolute risk for those aged 10 or more at the time of irradiation for all cancer excluding leukemia can be broken down into the respective sites as follows:

Type of Cancer	Deaths/10^6/year/rem
Breast	1.5*
Lung	1.3
GI incl. Stomach	1.0
Bone	0.2
All other cancer	1.0
Total	5.0

* This is derived from a value of 6.0 corrected for a 50% cure rate and the inclusion of males as well as females in the population.

TABLE 3

Estimated Risks of Radiation-Induced Cancer[a]

Type of Cancer	Population Affected	Lifetime cases per million per rem
Leukemia	A-bomb survivors; radiation therapy; thorotrast injections	10-60
Thyroid gland	A-bomb survivors; radiation therapy; Marshall Islanders	20-150
Breast (female)	A-bomb survivors; radiation therapy; multiple fluoroscopies	30-200
Lung	A-bomb survivors; radiation therapy; uranium miners	20-100
Bone	Radium ingestion and injection	5
Brain, salivary glands, stomach, liver, large intestine	A-bomb survivors; radiation therapy; thorotrast injections	10-15
Esophagus, small intestine, pancreas, rectum, bladder, ovary, lymphoid tissues, cranial sinuses, skin	A-bomb survivors; radiation therapy; radium ingestion	less than 5
	Total	100-1000

a From Nat. Acad. Sci., 1972; United Nations, 1977.

TABLE 4

Estimates of Annual Contribution of Radiation Exposure to
Lifetime Burden of Fatal Cancer to the U.S. Population[a]

(Total Cancer Mortality, 1975, 365,000)

Source	Lifetime cancer mortality commitment (Number of Deaths)
Natural Background	5,000
Technologically Enhanced Natural Radiation	250
Healing Arts	4,250
Nuclear Weapons Fallout	250–450
Occupational Irradiation	50–60
Nuclear Energy	9
Consumer Products	1.5
Total	<10,000
	= 2.7 percent of cancer mortality

[a] From Jablon and Bailar, 1980.

In the case of ultraviolet radiation from the sun, on
the other hand, the correlation between the incidence of skin
cancer and the intensity of exposure is clearly demonstrable
in fair-skinned populations (Fig. 12). Thus, with skin
cancer, the carcinogenic effects of sunlight at natural
background levels account for much of the natural occurrence
of this common form of cancer.

Because there is reason to think that the bulk of the
cancer burden is attributable to environmental factors yet to
be identifed, the challenge to press on with their identifca-
tion must not be neglected. Furthermore, since we cannot
hope to eliminate all carcinogens, a practical strategy for
cancer prevention will necessitate that we arrive at accept-
able risk-benefit assessments.

This approach will require increasingly close collaboration between epidemiologists and laboratory scientists.

Hence, we are fortunate this morning to begin our conference with a session concerning both the biology and the epidemiology of cancer.

REFERENCES

1. Boice, J.D., Land, C.E., Shore, R.E., Norman, J.E., and Tokunaga, M. Risk of breast cancer following low-dose radiation exposure. *Radiology 131:* 589-597, 1979.
2. Borek, C. In vitro cell transformation by low doses of X-irradiation and neutrons. In: Biology of Radiation Carcinogenesis, edited by J.M. Yuhas, R.W. Tennant, and J.D. Regan, Raven Press, New York, 1976, pp. 309-326.
3. Brown, J.M. The shape of the dose-response curve for radiation carcinogenesis. Extrapolation to low doses. *Radiat. Res. 71:* 34-50, 1977.
4. Cairns, J. The cancer problem. *Sci. Am. 233:*64-78,1975.
5. Cancer Facts and Figures. American Cancer Society, Inc., New York, 1980.
6. Doll, R. Strategy for the detection of cancer hazards to man. *Nature (London) 265:* 589-596, 1977.
7. Doll, R. An epidemiological perspective of the biology of cancer. *Cancer Res. 38:* 3573-3583, 1978.
8. Hirayama, T. Changing patterns of cancer in Japan with special reference to the decrease in stomach cancer mortality. In: Origins of Human Cancer, edited by H.H. Hiatt, J.D. Watson, and J.A. Winsten, Cold Spring Harbor Conference on Cell Proliferation, vol. 4, pp. 55-75, Cold Spring Harbor Laboratory, New York, 1977.
8. Ishimaru, T., Hoshino, T., Ichimaru, M., Okada, H., Tomiyasu, T., Tsuchimoto, T., and Yamamoto, T. Leukemia in the atomic bomb survivors of Hiroshima and Nagasaki, 1 October 1950-30 September 1966. *Radiat. Res. 45:* 216-233, 1971.
9. Jablon, S. and Bailar, J.A. The contribution of ionizing radiation to cancer mortality in the United States. *Preventive Medicine 9(2):* 219-226, 1980.
10. National Academy of Sciences. Advisory Committee on the Biological Effects of Ionizing Radiation. Effects on populations of exposure for low levels of ionizing radiation. National Academy of Sciences,Washington,1972.

11. Segi, M., Kurihara, M., and Matsuyama, T.   Cancer mortality for selected sites in 24 countries, No. 5, 1964-1965.   Dept. of Public Health, Tohoku University School of Medicine, Sendai, Japan, 1969.
12. Sparrow, A.H., Underbrin, A.G., and Rossi, H.H.   Mutations induced in tradescantia by small doses of X-rays and neutrons; analysis of dose-response curves. *Science 176:* 916-918, 1972.
13. Sugimura, T., Sato, S., Nagao, M., Yahagi, T., Matsushima, T., Seino, Y., Takeuchi, M., and Kawachi, T. Overlapping of carcinogens and mutagens.   In: Fundamentals in Cancer Prevention, edited by P.N. Magee, et al, Univ. of Tokyo Press, Tokyo/Univ. Park Press, Baltimore, 1976, pp. 191-215.
14. United Nations Scientific Committee on the Effects of Atomic Radiation.   Sources and Effects of Ionizing Radiation, Report to the General Assembly, with annexes, United Nations, New York, 1977.
15. Upton, A.C.   Progress in the prevention of cancer. *Preventive Medicine 7:* 476-485, 1978.

NATIONAL SURVEY OF CANCER MORTALITY
IN CHINA

LI PING AND LI JUN YAO
Cancer Institute
Chinese Academy of Medical Sciences
Beijing, China

Malignant diseases are a major threat to the health and
life of the people of China. Data on the incidence and
distribution of the common forms of cancer among the population are useful in studying carcinogenesis, organizing
prevention programs and evaluating cancer control activities.
Between 1975 and 1978, under a personal directive of our
beloved late Premier Zhou Enlai, health personnel mobilized
the masses for the purpose of conducting a nationwide cancer
mortality survey. The result has been a clarification of the
distribution of cancer mortality in China, and was reported
in the Atlas of Cancer Mortality in People's Republic of China
This provides a basis for future studies of cancer epidemiology and etiology. As indicated by the results of the survey,
cancer is one of the major causes of morbidity and mortality
among the Chinese people. This report presents findings of
the patterns and distribution of cancer in China.

MATERIALS AND METHODS

1. *SOURCE OF DATA*

In 1975, a three year survey was begun on the causes of
death in China. It was completed in 1978. Methods of
organization and execution of the survey are detailed elsewhere. Some of the results are published in the Atlas of
Cancer Mortality in the People's Republic of China. The
present report is based on the original data relating to the
total number of cancer deaths among the population on a sample
basis. The entire survey encompasses 29 provinces, municipalities and autonomous regions (395 cities and prefectures and
2101 counties), with a population of 850 million (Table 1).
Over a three year period, the number of deaths from cancer
among this population was determined. To compare the relation
of cancer deaths to other causes of deaths, calculations were
also made of other major causes of mortality.

TABLE 1.   AREAS SURVEYED FOR CAUSE OF DEATH IN CHINA

Administrative units	Total Number	Number Surveyed	%
Province Classification	30	29	96.7
Municipality	3	3	1oo.o
Province	22	21	95.5
Autonomous Region	5	5	1oo.o
Prefecture Classification	211	210	99.5
Prefecture	174	173	99.3
Autonomous State	29	29	1oo.o
Administrative District	1	1	1oo.o
League	7	7	1oo.o
City	185	185	1oo.o
County Classification	2136	2101	98.4
County (District)	2013	1978	98.3
Autonomous County	66	66	1oo.0
Banner	53	53	1oo.o
Autonomous Banner	3	3	1oo.o
Town	1	1	1oo.o

2. COMPLETENESS OF DATA

This three-year survey of cause of death encompasses all provinces, municipalities and autonomous regions in China except Taiwan province. Within the area of study, only the Ali prefecture in Tibet and a few counties in Sichuan were not investigated because of the vast area, sparse population and poor transportation. According to an official report in 1979, the population of China, including Taiwan, is 970 million. Of these, 850 million have been included in the three year survey, or a cumulative 2.5 billion person-years observation. Facts concerning the large majority of deaths among the population reported to residence registration stations are in accord with those of the present study.

3. RELIABILITY OF DATA

Among all patients in the study, 92.54% were diagnosed at commune-level facility at least, and 79.16% were seen at a county hospital or larger institution. Only 4.67% were seen only by barefoot doctors in production brigades. Another 2.79% were not seen by any medical personnel before death.

According to the methods used to make diagnoses, patients in this survey can be categorized into 4 groups. In Group I,

consisting of 16.66% of the survey patients, diagnosis ante-
mortem (histopathologic examination of tissue specimens, bone
marrow and cytology materials) was achieved. Group II, or
53.84%, was diagnosed by x-rays, endoscopy, exploratory examination without biopsy, immunologic tumor markers, ultrasound,
isotope scan or laboratory chemistry tests. These 2 groups
constitute 70.5% of all cancer patients surveyed. In Group
III, or 23.46% of the patients, diagnosis by clinical examination was made in 23.46% and the remaining 6.04% (Group IV)
was diagnosed retrospectively after death.

In addition, reliability of data is supported by the
facts that (1) repeat survey in a number of randomly selected
counties produced comparable results; (2) comparison with
other data on causes of death in regions with mortality registration showed the same findings; (3) there is consistence
with population screening data on esophageal cancer (using
exofoliative cytology), hepatoma (using alpha-feto-protein),
cervical cancer (cytology), nasopharyngeal carcinoma (by
inspection and biopsy), and lung cancer (chest film); (4)
comparable rates exist in adjoining geographic areas under
different provincial, municipal and autonomous regional juris-
diction.

Thus, the results of the present cancer mortality survey
are considered relatively reliable and usable in analyzing
cancer mortality patterns in China.

4. CLASSIFICATION OF CAUSES OF DEATH AND CANCER DEATH

The international system of disease classification was
adopted with attention to common medical conditions in China.
Deaths were classified into the following 20 major types: (1)
malignant neoplasms, (2) tuberculosis, (3) infectious diseases,
(4) parasitic diseases, (5) trauma, poisoning and accidents,
(6) nutritional deficiency, endocrine and metabolic diseases,
(7) diseases of blood and blood-forming organs, (8) psychia-
tric diseases, (9) diseases of the nervous system, (10) ar-
teriosclerotic heart disease, (11) other cardio-vascular
diseases, (12) cerebrovascular disease, (13) diseases of the
respiratory system, (14) diseases of the digestive system,
(15) diseases of the urinary and reproductive systems, (16)
diseases of pregnancy, delivery and postpartum periods, (17)
congenital anomalies, (18) neonatal diseases, (19) other
causes of death and (20) diagnosis unknown.

Deaths from malignant diseases were further divided into
15 categories not only according to anatomic sites but also
to pathologic features: (1) nasopharyngeal carcinoma, (2)
cancer of the esophagus, (3) cancer of the stomach, (4) cancer

of the liver, (5) cancer of the lung, (6) cancer of the
breast, (7) cancer of the uterine cervix, (8) leukemia, (9)
cancer of the colon and rectum, (10) cancer of the urinary
bladder, (11) cancer of the penis, (12) malignant lymphomas,
(13) choriocarcinoma, (14) brain tumors and (15) other malignant neoplasms.

5. STATISTICAL PROCEDURES

Statistical analyses of the cancer mortality survey were
made under the direction of a scientific and technical team.
Various statistical procedures utilized computer methods to
determine the distribution of cancer mortality by county,
prefecture, provinces, and country. Analyses included crude
mortality rate, age-adjusted mortality rate and cumulative
mortality rate. In calculating the age-adjusted mortality
rate, three standard populations were used: population of
China (age composition of the 1964 population), world population; and truncated population, ages 35 to 64, of the world.
The results are the age-adjusted cancer mortality rates
standardized to the population of China, the world population
and truncated world population. Because of inadequacies of
data for persons over 75, cumulative mortality rates for age
groups 0 to 64 and 0 to 74 were calculated (expressed as
percentages) to show the cumulative cancer mortality probability up to the ages of 65 and 75.

6. METHODS OF GROUPING AND RANKING OF DATA

To compare and contrast the epidemiologic features of
cancer in China, the following statistical methods were employed to group and rank the mortality data.
(1) Ranking by percentile. The geographic units studied
were ranked in the order of their cancer mortality rate,
assigned a percentile ranking and reported by the appropriate
decile rank.
(2) Ranking by geometric gradient. Formula 2 (n-2) was
used, yielding grades at levels of 0.5, 2, 4, 16, 32, 64, 128
and 256 deaths per 100,000.
(3) Ranking by statistical significance test. The age-
adjusted mortality rate for each geographic area of study was
compared with the age adjusted national rate to determine
those areas showing a statistically significant difference.
The mortality rate data were then sorted into five levels.
(4) Division by major age groups. Rates were determined
for five major age groups: children, 0 to 14 years; young
adults, 15 to 34 years; middle age, 35 to 54 years; elderly,

55 to 74 and 75 years and over.

(5) Grading by urban-rural gradient. Rates in urban and rural areas were compared. In addition, cities were divided into three grades: large cities (750,000), medium-sized cities (250,000 to 750,000) and small cities (less than 250,000). Comparison of urban and rural areas employed data for 157 cities of diverse sizes and 307 randomly selected rural counties.

(6) Division by nationalities. This was made for the following minorities according to autonomous regions, autonomous counties or banners: Mongol, Hui, Zhuang, Uygur, Miao, Yi, Korean and Kezak.

RESULTS AND DISCUSSION

1. THREAT OF MALIGNANT DISEASES

(1) Major causes of deaths in China

From 1973 to 1975, among males, cancer was the second leading cause of mortality. It was the third leading cause of death among females. Cancer was the cause of 11.31% of deaths among males and 8.85% of deaths among females. The burden of cancer varied with age. Among children of 0 to 14 years, cancer accounted for 0.80% of deaths and ranked eleventh among causes of death, whereas among people of 35 to 54 years of age, cancer became the leading cause of death (21.58%) (Tables 2 and 3). This shows that cancer is a significant cause of death, particularly among the working age groups. In China, cancer is the leading cause of death among males in Shanghai, Jiangsu, Fujian, Zhejiang and among females in Jiangsu. Cancer is the second leading cause of deaths among males in Henan, Shanxi, Hebei, Anhui, Shaanxi, Jilin, Liaoning and Shandong, and among females in Shanghai, Fujian, Zhejiang and Shandong. It is third in Beijing, Tienjin, Chinghai, Inner-Mongolia, Heilongjiang, among males; and in Shanxi, Shaanxi, Inner Mongolia, Tienjin and Beijing among females. Cancer is among the three leading causes of death among males in 17 provinces, municipalities, and autonomous regions, and among females in ten. Cancer is the leading cause of death among males in 60 prefectures (cities) and among females in 21; it is second among males in 38 prefectures (cities) and among females in 25. Cancer is the leading cause of death among males in 429 counties or equivalent areas and among females in 161. It is second among males in 259 counties and among females in 202. It is third among males in 277 counties and among females in 357.

TABLE 2.   PROPORTIONAL MORTALITY RATES OF THE TOTAL
POPULATION IN BROAD AGE
GROUPS IN CHINA 1973-1977

Cause of death (0---)	%	Cause of death (15---)	%	Cause of death (35---)	%
1. Respiratory diseases	19.43	1. Trauma poisoning and accidents	25.71	1. Cancer	21.58
2. Neonatal diseases	17.81	2. Tuberculosis	9.87	2. Other heart-vascular diseases	12.84
3. Infectious diseases	16.03	3. Other heart-vascular diseases	8.05	3. Tuberculosis	10.27
4. Trauma poisoning and accidents	12.33	4. Cancer	7.88	4. Digestive diseases	9.06
5. Digestive diseases	6.44	5. Infectious diseases	6.56	5. Trouma, poisoning and accidents	8.42
6. Other heart-vascular diseases	1.82	6. Digestive diseases	5.09	6. Respiratory diseases	5.01
7. Endocrine, nutritional deficiency and metabolic diseases	1.60	7. Pregnancy-related diseases	3.77	7. Cerebrovascular diseases	4.55
8. Tuberculosis	1.26	8. Urinary diseases	2.34	8. Infectious diseases	3.07
9. Congenital anomalies	1.04	9. Psychosis	1.64	9. Arteriosclerotic heart diseases	2.18
10. Urinary diseases	0.83	10. Nervous system diseases	1.52	10. Urinary diseases	1.83

TABLE 3.   PROPORTIONAL MORTALITY RATES OF THE TOTAL
POPULATION IN BROAD AGE
GROUPS IN CHINA 1973-1977

Cause of death (55---)	%	Cause of death (75---)	%
1. Other heart-vascular diseases	17.39	1. Other heart-vascular diseases	16.27
2. Cancer	16.09	2. Respiratory diseases	15.66
3. Respiratory diseases	11.29	3. Cerebrovascular diseases	14.57
4. Cerebrovascular diseases	10.85	4. Digestive diseases	7.29
5. Digestive diseases	7.45	5. Arteriosclerotic heart diseases	6.12
6. Tuberculosis	5.85	6. Cancer	5.96
7. Arteriosclerotic heart disease	4.00	7. Infectious diseases	4.10
8. Trauma, poisoning and accidents	3.09	8. Tuberculosis	2.43
9. Infectious diseases	2.60	9. Urinary diseases	1.91
10. Urinary diseases	1.72	10. Trauma, poisoning and accidents	0.68

(2) Number of cancer deaths per year

Among the population of 900 million in China, approximately 700,000 die of cancer each year, or one every 40 seconds. There are 160,000 deaths from gastric cancer, 157,000 from esophageal cancer, and 100,000 from liver cancer. These are the three leading causes of cancer mortality. The highest number of deaths are in Jiangsu (about 70,000), Henan (about 60,000), Shandong (about 50,000) and Sichuan (about 50,000).

(3) Cancer mortality rate

In China, the cancer mortality rate (age-adjusted to standard world population) is 99.46 per 100,000; it is 119.64/100,000 in males and 80.69/100,000 in females. Comparison with worldwide data shows that although rates in China are lower than in the industrialized nations of Europe and North America, the figures are higher than in the developing countries. There are 13 provinces, municipalities and autonomous regions in China in which the sex-specific mortality adjusted to the world Standard exceeds 100/100,000. In a few of these areas, the cancer mortality rate exceeds the highest world rates (Figure 1).

(4) Cumulative cancer mortality rate

The cumulative cancer mortality rate from 0 to 74 years of age is 14.74% among males, and 9.45% among females. It is lower than that of Europe, North America and Australia, but higher than that of some developing countries. The cumulative mortality rate in some provinces approaches and even exceeds the highest figures among other nations. In Shanghai, for example, the figure is between 20 and 25% among males, or one-fourth to one-fifth of all deaths. Yang Zhong County in Jiangsu has the highest cumulative mortality rate in China. Its cumulative mortality rate (age 0-74 years) is 52.18% among males and 40.21% among females. The figures show that through 74 years of age, nearly one-half of the population die of cancer.

FIGURE 1

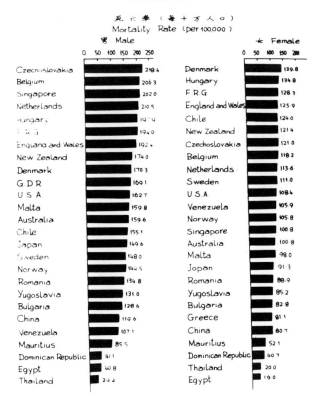

死亡率（每十万人口）
Mortality Rate (per 100,000)

男 Male

女 Female

	0 50 100 150 200 250				0 50 100 150 200	
Czechoslovakia	218.4		Denmark	139.8
Belgium	206.3		Hungary	134.8
Singapore	202.0		F.R.G.	128.3
Netherlands	210.5		England and Wales	125.9
Hungary	197.4		Chile	124.0
F.R.G.	194.0		New Zealand	121.4
England and Wales	192.4		Czechoslovakia	121.0
New Zealand	174.0		Belgium	118.2
Denmark	170.3		Netherlands	113.6
G.D.R.	169.1		Sweden	111.0
U.S.A.	162.7		U.S.A.	108.4
Malta	159.8		Venezuela	105.9
Australia	159.6		Norway	105.8
Chile	155.1		Singapore	100.8
Japan	149.6		Australia	100.8
Sweden	148.0		Malta	98.0
Norway	144.5		Japan	91.3
Romania	134.8		Romania	88.9
Yugoslavia	131.0		Yugoslavia	85.2
Bulgaria	128.6		Bulgaria	82.8
China	119.6		Greece	81.1
Venezuela	107.1		China	80.7
Mauritius	85.5		Mauritius	52.1
Dominican Republic	41.1		Dominican Republic	40.7
Egypt	40.8		Thailand	20.0
Thailand	22.2		Egypt	19.0

世界部分国家和地区恶性肿瘤年龄调整死亡率
Age-adjusted Mortality Rates for Malignant
Neoplasms in Selected Countries

50

(5)   Average death-age of cancer cases

    The average age at death from cancer in China is 58.15
years (Table 4).   The ages were 57.71 for males and 58.75 for
females.   By site, urinary bladder cancer shows the highest
average age at death (65.70 years), and is followed by
esophageal cancer (63.49) and cancer of the penis (62.80
years).   The lowest average age is for leukemia (27.16 years),
and brain tumors (40.66 years).   More than 60% of cancer
deaths occur in persons between 20 and 64 years of age; cancer
is an important cause of death among the working population.

TABLE 4.   AVERAGE DEATH-AGE OF CANCER CASES IN CHINA (YEARS)

SITE	MALE	FEMALE	TOTAL
Stomach	61.11	62.59	61.62
Esophagus	63.04	64.31	63.49
Liver	53.71	57.59	54.83
Cervix Uteri	————	58.96	58.96
Lung	59.50	59.68	59.56
Colon/Rectum	59.03	60.36	59.60
Leukemia	26.94	28.09	27.16
Nasophrynx	52.27	54.74	53.12
Breast	62.70	57.80	57.91
Brain	46.33	41.11	40.66
Lymphoma	48.49	52.06	49.99
Bladder	66.01	64.85	65.70
Penis	62.80	————	62.80
Choriocarcinoma	————	41.18	41.18
Total	57.71	58.75	58.15

(6)   Cancer mortality by anatomic site

    Cancers of the upper alimentary tract are most common.
Stomach cancer is the most common neoplasm in China.   It
accounts for 26.11% of cancer deaths in men and 18.72% in
women.   Esophageal cancer is the second leading cause of
cancer deaths in men, accounting for 24.55% of all cancer
deaths.   Liver cancer ranks third.   About 60% of all cancer
deaths was due to cancers of the digestive tract.   Cancer of
the uterine cervix, lung, colon and rectum, leukemia, nasopharynx and breast also displayed high rates.   These nine
primary cancers account for 90% of all cancer deaths (table 5).

TABLE 5.   CANCER MORTALITY RATES* BY SITE AND SEX IN CHINA
(1973-1977)

Site	Rate	MALE %	Site	Rate	FEMALE %
Stomach	20.93	26.11	Stomach	10.16	18.72
Esophagus	19.68	24.55	Cervix Uteri	9.98	18.39
Liver	14.52	18.11	Esophagus	9.85	18.15
Lung	6.82	8.51	Liver	5.61	10.34
Colon/Rectum	4.08	5.09	Lung	3.20	5.90
Leukemia	2.79	3.48	Colon/Rectum	3.03	5.58
Nasopharynx	2.49	3.11	Breast	2.61	4.81
Brain	1.43	1.78	Leukemia	2.23	4.11
Lymphoma	1.35	1.68	Nasopharynx	1.27	2.34
Bladder	0.80	1.00	Brain	1.07	1.97
Penis	0.39	0.49	Lymphoma	0.96	1.77
Breast	0.06	0.07	Bladder	0.27	0.50
Other	4.83	6.03	Choriocarcinoma	0.23	0.42
			Other	3.80	7.00
Total	80.17	100.00	Total	54.27	100.00

* Age-adjusted to population in China, 1964.

2.   DISTRIBUTION OF CANCER IN THE POPULATION

(1) By sex. In China, as in most parts of the world,
cancer mortality is higher in males. The sex ratio of the
mortality rate of cancer, adjusted to the world population
is 1.48 (M:F). The sex ratio differs among nationalities,
and is lowest for the Uygur minority (1.05) and highest for
the Koreans (1.76). The sex ratios are highest for urinary
bladder cancer (2.96), liver cancer (2.59), lung cancer (2.13)
gastric cancer (2.06) and esophageal cancer (2.00). The
lowest ratios are for breast cancer (0.02), leukemia (1.25)
and colorectal cancer (1.34).

(2) By age. The cancer mortality rates are lowest in the
5 to 14 year age group and rise thereafter. The rise is
greatest at ages 35 to 39 years. After 75 years of age, the
rate declines among males but not among females.

The mortality rates and cancer sites vary with age. Among children ages 0 to 14 years, leukemia is commonest and comprise 52.91% of all malignancies. Other common cancers in children are brain tumors and lymphomas. Among young adults (ages 15 to 34) the commonest cancer is liver cancer (18.81%). Leukemia is also common (20.86%). Among more elderly persons, however, gastric, esophageal, liver and lung cancers predominate (Table 6).

The age curves for individual sites of cancer in China display noteworthy features. One pattern is represented by cancers of the esophagus, stomach, lung, colon and rectum, bladder and penis. These cancers rise in frequency with age. A second pattern is represented by cancer of the uterine cervix. It is most common in the middle ages, and decline in frequency in the elderly. The third pattern is represented by breast cancer which rapidly rises in frequency in early adulthood and more slowly after 45 years of age. A fourth pattern is seen in liver cancer and nasopharyngeal cancer. These rise in frequency after adolescence, continue to rise in adulthood and remain high in frequency in the elderly. A fifth pattern is seen in acute leukemia which peaks in frequency in children, declines thereafter, and has stable rates in adulthood. A sixth pattern is seen in gestational choriocarcinoma, which occurs primarily in the childbearing ages. Analyses of the age patterns of specific cancers can provide etiologic clues. Furthermore, analyses of age patterns of cancer by geographic area can suggest the role of localized carcinogenic influences.

(3) <u>By nationality</u>. In China, cancer rates are highest in the Kazak (111.24/100,000), the Hui (85.74) and the Korean (71.32) national minorities. The Miao and Yi have the lowest rates (30.14 and 32.35). As a fractional representation of all deaths, cancer is highest among the Kazak (14.87%), the Koreans (10.33%) and the Hui (9.44%). The lowest is in the Miao (2.83%). The cumulative mortality rates display comparable patterns. Differences in cancer mortality among nationalities may be due to differences in living environment. But lifestyle may also account for these differences. For example, both the Kazak and Uygur live in Sinjiang in close geographic proximity; however, the Kazak have a cancer mortality rate twice that of the Uygur (111.24 versus 53.72/100,000). Although mortality of cancers of the stomach, uterine cervix, esophagus, liver and lung is high in all nationalities, the rates are substantially different. For example, gastric cancer mortality is highest in males of all nationalities, but the age adjusted mortality, standardized

TABLE 6. MORTALITY RATES* AND PROPORTION FOR THE FIVE
LEADING CANCER SITES IN MAJOR AGE GROUPS,
CHINA (1973-1977)

UNDER 15	15---34	35---54	55---74	75 +
Leukemia 2.33 (52.91%)	Leukemia 2.44 (20.86%)	Liver 23.33 (21.36%)	Esophagus 114.63 (26.99%)	Esophagus 183.78 (30.20%)
Brain 0.55 (12.50%)	Liver 2.20 (18.81%)	Stomach 22.83 (20.89%)	Stomach 113.83 (26.64%)	Stomach 155.26 (25.52%)
Lymphoma 0.31 (7.05%)	Stomach 0.98 (8.41 %)	Esophagus 17.92 (16.40%)	Liver 52.04 (12.25%)	Colon/Rectum 47.23 (7.77%)
Liver 0.18 (4.17%)	Brain 0.87 (7.43%)	Cervix 9.82 (8.99%)	Lung 34.40 (8.10%)	Liver 47.10 (7.74%)
Nasopharynx 0.05 (1.11%)	Colon/Rectum 0.77 (6.66%)	Lung 8.44 (7.74%)	Cervix 31.92 (7.52%)	Cervix 39.00 (6.41%)

* per 100,000 population,

TABLE 7. AGE-ADJUSTED MORTALITY RATES (PER 100,000) FOR CANCER BY MINORITY NATIONALITY IN CHINA (MALE)

Site	Monggol	Hui	Zang	Uygur	Miao	Yi	Korean	Kazak
Stomach	23.27	50.65	29.45	18.21	7.82	11.42	31.71	48.26
Esophagus	12.89	18.90	7.80	12.87	1.61	1.67	5.82	39.27
Liver	10.43	13.30	10.32	7.07	7.73	8.66	22.75	15.29
Lung	6.25	3.85	2.04	4.15	2.53	1.96	11.32	5.78
Colon/Rectum	4.36	3.55	2.86	2.81	2.50	2.27	3.60	3.60
Leukemia	2.75	2.78	1.72	1.92	1.71	2.15	3.12	2.46
Nasopharynx	1.19	1.15	0.98	1.01	3.04	1.81	1.48	0.55
Brain	1.69	1.33	1.46	1.01	0.93	0.79	1.66	1.49
Lymphoma	1.40	1.33	0.75	1.15	1.05	0.88	1.17	1.61
Bladder	0.92	1.21	0.38	0.39	0.52	0.28	1.35	1.41
Penis	0.35	0.17	0.06	0.13	0.39	0.14	0.28	0.17
Other	4.25	5.91	4.14	4.21	3.79	3.19	6.96	7.51
Total	69.79	104.09	61.89	54.95	33.62	35.23	91.17	127.36

TABLE 8. AGE-ADJUSTED MORTALITY RATES (PER 10^{-5}) FOR CANCER BY MINORITY IN CHINA (FEMALE)

Site	Monggol	Hui	Zang	Uygur	Miao	Yi	Korean	Kazak
Stomach	12.03	22.43	18.91	10.31	5.43	8.22	15.40	26.56
Cervix Uteri	15.72	12.29	4.84	17.27	5.51	5.16	8.41	9.67
Esophagus	5.73	6.32	5.34	7.93	0.63	0.91	1.62	27.08
Liver	4.75	5.82	5.66	3.70	3.29	3.47	6.68	7.82
Lung	1.73	2.22	1.29	1.90	1.21	1.26	4.89	2.58
Colon/Rectum	3.61	2.81	1.65	2.15	1.66	1.84	2.56	2.57
Breast	2.72	1.99	1.25	1.65	1.53	1.76	2.51	2.68
Leukemia	2.65	2.05	0.78	1.72	1.06	0.96	2.68	1.91
Nasopharynx	0.80	0.70	0.33	0.45	1.73	0.69	0.42	0.41
Brain	1.28	1.29	0.97	0.85	0.57	0.50	0.89	1.05
Lymphoma	0.83	1.06	0.53	0.89	0.78	0.65	0.94	1.13
Bladder	0.25	0.51	0.14	0.17	0.16	0.00	0.24	0.31
Choriocarcinoma	0.22	0.32	0.37	0.14	0.33	0.48	0.08	0.25
Other	3.81	4.58	3.97	3.01	2.78	3.83	4.55	6.54
Total	57.07	64.40	46.04	52.18	26.71	29.71	51.78	90.67

to the Chinese population shows wide variance. The Kazak
and the Hui nationalities have the highest age-adjusted rates
of gastric cancer (48.26 and 50.56/100,000), which are five
to six times those of the Miao and Yi nationalities, which
have the lowest rates of gastric cancer (7.82 and 11.42/
100,000 respectively). Among females, the differences are
more striking. The Hui, Korean, Zang, and Yi die of gastric
cancer most frequently; Uygur, Mongol, and Miao die of cancer
of the uterine cervix most frequently. Among the Kazak,
esophageal cancer ranks first (Tables 7,8).

Age and sex-specific cancer mortality rates show variation among nationalities. Uterine cervix cancer mortality
is high among young women. As a result the Mongols, ages
30 to 44, and the Uygur, age 25, show an overall mortality
rate from cancer higher in females than in males.

3.   GEOGRAPHIC DISTRIBUTION OF CANCER

(1) Distribution by province, municipality and autonomous
     region

The provinces, municipalities and autonomous regions in
China show differences in cancer mortality rates. In coastal,
northern and northwestern China, cancer mortality is relatively high. It is lower in south and southwest China (Fig.2)
In 12 provinces, municipalities and autonomous regions, the
rates exceed the national rate. Among them, the areas with
crude cancer mortality rates over 100/100,000 and age-
adjusted rate over 80/100,000 are Jiangsu, Shanghai, Fujien,
Ningxia, Zhejiang, Shanxi. The crude mortality rate is
highest in Shanghai (140.66/100,000), which is 3.52 times
higher than that in Yunnan (31.0). The age-adjusted rate
(China's standard) is highest in Jiangsu (101.56), which is
2.43 times higher than that in Yunnan (29.63). Among males,
in 17 provinces, municipalities and autonomous regions,
gastric cancer mortality ranks first. It comprises between
19.53% and 57.51% of all cancers (highest in Chinghai). In
nine other areas, esophageal cancer is most common, compris-
ing between 20.87% and 45.10% (highest in Henan) of cancers.
In three provinces, liver cancer is commonest: Hunan, Guangdong and Guangxi. In Guangxi the proportion is 48.84%. The
second and third commonest cancers are also gastric, liver,
or esophageal in most instances. However, nasopharyngeal
cancer is third in Guangdong and Guangxi. In Shanghai,
Beijing, Yunnan, and the northeastern provinces, lung cancer
is third. Among females, several cancers are among the
highest in frequency. Gastric cancer is most frequent in
11 areas and cervical cancer is commonest in eight.

FIGURE 2

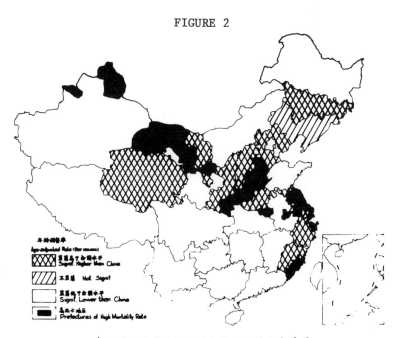

中国男性恶性肿瘤高死亡率地区地理分布图
Geographic Distribution of Areas of High Mortality Rate for Malignant Neoplasms in China

Esophageal cancer is commonest in seven others, lung cancer
is commonest in Beijing and Tienjin, and liver cancer is
commonest in Guangxi.   The second most common is cervical
cancer in 15 areas, gastric cancer in nine, liver cancer in
Guangdong, Shanghai, Tibet, and esophageal cancer in Shansi
and Hubei.

(2) Distribution of cancer mortality by county

      The distribution of cancer rates in the 2392 counties
(age-adjusted to the Chinese population standard) was studied.
The rates for males range between 9.75-279.33/100,000 and
for females between 6.90-213.64/100,000. For each decile,
the rates are higher in males than in females. The age-
adjusted mortality rates were compared with the national rate.
Statistically significant elevations in rates are found for
males in 28.01% of the counties and for females in 30.14%.
No significant differences from the national rate are found
for males in 20.53% of the counties, and for females in 28.05%.
Significantly lower rates are found for males in the

remaining 51.46% of the counties, and for females in 41.81%.
    The adjusted mortality rates for cancer among counties
were examined for distribution by a geometric gradient of
rates. For males 42.43% of the counties have rates below
64/100,000, and 10.70% had rates exceeding 128/100,000. In
females, 70.11% of the counties have rates below 64.0/100,000
and 29.89% have rates above 64/100,000. Only 2.17% exceed
128/100,000.

(3) Distribution of cancer by urban-rural areas

    Cancer mortality rates differ in rural and urban areas.
In general, cities have higher rates, with highest rates in
the largest cities. Rural-urban differences are also seen
for the proportion of total deaths that are due to cancer.
However, differences related to sex are small. Analysis by
site shows the highest mortality rate for stomach cancer in
cities, and for esophageal cancer in rural areas. The
second commonest is lung cancer in large cities, esophageal
cancer in medium and small cities, and gastric cancer in
rural areas. In cities as well as in rural areas, liver
cancer is third in frequency. In addition to differences
in the order of frequency, rural-urban differences in
mortality rates are also seen. Lung, stomach, liver and
urinary bladder cancers are relatively more common in urban
areas. Among females, breast cancers, colorectal cancer,
leukemia, brain tumors and lymphomas are more common in
urban areas. The urban excess is greatest for lung cancer,
followed by liver cancer. The marked predominance of these
cancers in large cities is perhaps due to different stan-
dards of living, overcrowding, pollution and urban lifestyles.
Rural areas have higher rates of esophageal and cervical
cancer mortality. Part of the gradient may be due to better
medical facilities in cities and the resultant lower case-
fatality rates; hygienic and dietary habits and standard of
living may be contributing factors.
    Age-specific data show, in general, higher cancer
mortality rates among urban populations, particularly among
the young and the elderly. However, in the working age
population rural rates are higher. The distribution of
urban-rural patterns are useful in studies of etiologic
factors. (Table 9).

TABLE 9.   URBAN-RURAL DIFFERENCES IN
MORTALITY OF CANCER OF
SELECTED SITES IN CHINA

Site	Age-adjusted Rate Urban (City)			Rural
	Large	Inter mediate	Small	
Stomach	21.38	22.04	21.87	23.20
Esophagus	13.11	21.16	18.87	24.78
Liver	14.48	14.20	14.64	14.31
Cervix Uteri	5.42	6.27	7.17	7.39
Lung	16.17	11.70	10.21	6.21
Intestine	5.79	4.98	5.48	5.29
Lleukemia	3.89	3.86	3.83	3.76
Nasopharynx	1.80	1.87	2.41	2.18
Breast	2.44	2.11	2.27	1.81
Brain	2.17	1.85	2.14	1.64
Lymphoma	1.73	1.56	1.56	1.66
Bladder	1.23	0.82	1.10	0.69
Penis	0.17	0.19	0.14	0.28
Choriocarcinoma	0.07	0.07	0.10	0.18
Other	10.15	7.36	8.21	6.62
All	100.00	100.00	100.00	100.00

(4)   Patterns of major cancers in China by geographic
characteristics

The relation of geographic characteristics to the distribution patterns of cancer in China is reported in the

Atlas of Cancer Maps of the People's Republic of China. The
maps show substantial variations in cancer patterns according to geography. Some cancers are common throughout China;
Others are more prevalent in some parts of China and much
less in other parts. These patterns are useful in carcinogenesis studies and cancer control activities.

1. Stomach cancer

The high mortality rate areas are in northwestern and
coastal China. The areas involved include Gansu, Chinghai,
Ningxi, Shanghai, Jiangsu, Zhejiang, Fujien, and the Liadong
and Shandong Peninsulas.

2. Cancer of the esophagus

Areas with a concentration of esophageal cancer can be
found within short distances from areas with much lower
rates. Concentric gradients of esophageal cancer are dis-
cernable between high and low rate areas. Differences among
the nationalities are also evident, as among the Kazaks. The
major high mortality rate areas are: (1) border area of the
three northern Chinese provinces (Hubei, Henan and Shansi),
(2) northern Sichuan, (3) the Dabie Mountain area of Hubei,
Henan and Anhui, (4) the northeastern area of Guangdong and
the south of Fujien, (5) northern Jiangsu and (6) areas
occupied by the Kazaks in Singiang.

3. Liver cancer

High cancer mortality areas are concentrated in the
southeastern coastal provinces and northeast Jilin. The
areas involved include Guangdong, Guangxi, Fujien, Zhejiang,
Shanghai, Jiangsu, Jilin, and particularly the coastal areas
of southeast China reaching to areas with gradually lower
rates in the interior. Highest rates are found in Fusui in
Grangxi and Qidong in Jiangsu.

4. Cancer of the uterine cervix

Rates are generally higher in rural areas. The adjoining high rate areas are Inner-Mongolia, Shanxi, Shaanxi,
Hubei, Hunan and Jianxi. The highest rates are in western
Hubei, south Shaanxi, southeast Shanxi, and the border
between Hunan and Jiangxi. The Uygur and Mongol nationalities show differences in mortality rates.

5. Lung cancer

Rates are generally higher in urban areas. The high
rate areas include Shanghai, Tienjin and Beijing, the three
northeast provinces, and the coastal areas of Jiangsu and
Zhejiang. These areas are industrialized, suggesting an

etiologic role of industrial development. In the three
northeastern provinces of China, the rates are high in both
males and females. Heating of homes during the long winter
and the smoking habits of women may be additional etiologic
factors, as well as those attributed to industry. Lung
cancer is uncommon in southwestern China, though the rates
are relatively high in Gejou city in Yunnan province (males)
and in Xuenwei (females).

6. Cancer of the colon and rectum

The high-rate areas are Zhejiang, Fujien, Jiangsu,
Shanghai, and areas near the lower reaches of the Yangtze
River. This region was the endemic area for schistomiasis
in China. Also, northern and northeastern China have some
high rate areas, but the geographic distribution shows no
striking patterns.

7. Leukemia

High rate areas are in eastern, northern, and northeastern provinces, such as Jiangsu, Fujien, and Shanghai.
In general, rates are higher in urban than in rural areas.

8. Nasopharyngeal carcinoma

High mortality rate areas encompass the south China
provinces of Guangdong, Guangxi, Hunan and Jiangsi, etc.
There is a gradient of rates from south (high) to north (low).
In Guangdong, the regions of Zhao Ching, Fushan and Guangzhou
have particularly high rates. Among the nationalities the
cancer is seen most among the Miao.

9. Breast cancer

The patterns of breast cancer are comparable to those
of lung cancer. In Beijing, Tienjin and Shanghai, northeast
China, and Liaoning, Jilin and other northern provinces, the
disease occurs more frequently. Rates are generally higher
in cities particularly large cities. However, no outstanding differences by geographic region are seen.

10. Urinary bladder cancer

Urinary bladder cancer patterns also resemble those for
lung cancer, with the highest rates in cities. The sex ratio
(M:F) is highest among the common cancers in China. The
areas with high mortality rates include Beijing, Tienjin,
Shanghai, and the areas of northern and northeastern China.

4.   DISTRIBUTION OF REGIONS WITH HIGH CANCER MORTALITY RATES

(1) Cancer as a major cause (among the first three) of death
     at the county level

Among 25 provinces, municipalities and autonomous
regions, cancer is the leading cause of death among males in
21.9% of counties and among females in 8.2%; cancer is second
among males in 13.2% of counties and among females in 10.3%;
cancer is third among males in 14% of counties and among
females in 18.1%. Cancer is among the three leading causes
of death in males in 49.1% of counties and in females in
36.6%.

(2) Cities, prefectures, counties with high age-adjusted
     mortality rates of cancer

The mortality rates of cities, prefectures, and counties
were ranked in order. Those with age-adjusted rates that
are 1.5 times (for cities and prefectures) or two times (for
counties) the national rate were selected and were considered
high rate units (for cities and prefectures, a cancer mortality rate exceeding 120/100,000 among males and 80/100,000
among females, and for counties a mortality rate exceeding
160/100,000 among males and 108/100,000 among females, with
adequate number of inhabitants to provide stable figures for
statistical analyses.

(3) Regions with high mortality rates due to the major
     forms of cancer in China

To assist responsible agencies in their carcinogenesis
studies and cancer prevention work, we arranged in order the
mortality rate for each of the common cancers in the 2392
counties in China. The highest one percent were selected
as high rate counties. Identification of these high rate
areas are useful in studies of cancer etiology and epidemiologic investigations of distribution patterns.

SUMMARY

A nation-wide retrospective survey of cancer mortality
for a three-year period was conducted in China. It covered
395 cities and 2136 counties with a population of more than
850 million. Data were collected on mortality from 56 causes
including 15 types of cancers. They were subjected to repeated scrutiny, and were considered reliable. Cancer was
found to be the second and third leading causes of death
among males and females, respectively. It was the leading

cause of death in 429 counties among males and in 161
counties among females. Approximately 700,000 people died
of cancer each year in China, with a crude mortality rate of
73.99 per 100,000. There were 13 provinces in China in which
the cancer mortality rate (age-adjusted to the world standard
population) exceeded 100 per 100,000. By anatomic site,
cancers of the upper alimentary tract were most common.
Stomach cancer was the commonest while esophageal cancer
ranked second and liver cancer third in frequency. These
three cancers accounted for 60% of all cancer deaths. By
nationality, cancer rates were highest in the Kazak, the Hui
and the Korean national minorities. The Miao and Yi had the
lowest rates. Some cancers were common throughout China,
whereas others displayed remarkable distribution by geographical areas. These geographical characteristics are to
be reported in the Atlas of Cancer Mortality in the People's
Republic of China. The national survey has provided us with
a better knowledge of cancer incidence, its distribution in
China and with a solid basis for cancer control in the years
to come.

GEOGRAPHIC PATTERNS OF CANCER
IN THE UNITED STATES

WILLIAM J. BLOT AND JOSEPH F. FRAUMENI, JR.
Environmental Epidemiology Branch
National Cancer Institute

Clues to the origins of cancer may come from case clusters of disease occurring among small groups over short periods of time[1]. Thus, a few cases of hepatic angiosarcoma among workers in Louisville, Kentucky, led to the identification of vinyl chloride as the responsible agent[2]. A cluster of vaginal adenocarcinoma among young women in Boston was traced to synthetic estrogens that were taken by their mothers during pregnancy[3]. In both situations the cancer in question was extremely rare in the general population so that the occurrence of even a few cases raised suspicion. Clustering of more common tumors is not obvious through clinical experience, but may be detected through a systematic monitoring of cancer morbidity and mortality statistics.

GEOGRAPHIC APPROACH

This paper reviews some epidemiologic studies at the National Cancer Institute that have utilized routinely collected mortality data to generate cancer statistics at the county level. Our investigations have involved a step-wise approach. First, using mortality data for 1950-1969, age-adjusted rates were calculated by sex and race for 35 cancers for each of the 3056 counties of the U.S., and the distribution of these rates was plotted in a series of computer-generated maps[4-6]. The geographic clusters and patterns were often unexpected and dramatic. For some of the common tumors, the maps have been updated to cover deaths through 1975.

Secondly, the county cancer rates have been correlated with demographic industrial, and environmental data available at the county level, in efforts to explore and refine the etiologic hypotheses that may help explain the geographic pecularities.

Finally, we have embarked upon field studies in various parts of the U.S. with elevated mortality rates. These are mostly case-control studies, in which individuals with and without a particular cancer are interviewed for lifetime histories of residence, occupation, smoking, and other suspected risk factors. Comparisons between cancer cases and controls are then made in an attempt to identify the environmental exposures responsible for the high cancer rates in a given area.

SKIN CANCER

One of the first maps we prepared dealt with skin cancer other than melanoma, which showed elevated mortality rates throughout the southern U.S. (Figure 1). The major cause of skin cancer is exposure to mid-wave ultraviolet radiation (UV-B) from sunlight. Since sunlight exposure is greatest in duration and intensity in the South, the map fits the expected pattern. This was of special interest at the time, since few people who develop skin cancer die from it. Although the map was based on a small fraction of incident cases, the clear geographic pattern suggested that the county mortality system was robust in reflecting carcinogenic exposures, and that the maps for other kinds of cancer may produce meaningful clues. Although sunlight exposure is related less clearly to skin melanoma, the distribution of melanoma showed a latitudinal gradient resembling that seen for other skin cancers.

RESPIRATORY CANCER

The maps for lung cancer showed some unexpected patterns. Mortality was high in New York, New Jersey and the urban northeast, but even higher in certain seaboard areas in the South. Clusters of elevated rates were seen along the Gulf Coast from Texas to the Florida panhandle, and along the southeast Atlantic coast from Virginia to northern Florida. Along with the temporal variations in lung cancer, there has been a shift in geographic distribution. As shown in Figure 2, the rate of increase in mortality from 1950-1975 has been faster in the southeast than in the northeast, for both urban and rural counties. Areas of high mortality are now primarily in the South as indicated by the updated map of lung cancer rates for 1970-1975 (Figure 3). Whereas 16% of northeast counties ranked in the upper decile in the early 1950's, only 2% were so ranked in the early 1970's.

Cigarette smoking is primarily responsible for the rising incidence of lung cancer in the U.S. and other nations. National surveys have shown that people in cities tend to smoke more than those on farms, accounting for part of the urban excess of lung cancer. Furthermore, northeasterners are said to be giving up smoking in greater numbers than

Figure 1

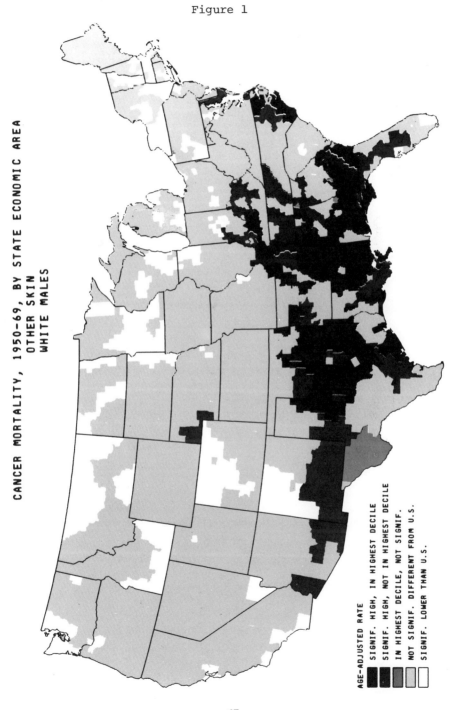

CANCER MORTALITY, 1950-69, BY STATE ECONOMIC AREA
OTHER SKIN
WHITE MALES

AGE-ADJUSTED RATE

SIGNIF. HIGH, IN HIGHEST DECILE

SIGNIF. HIGH, NOT IN HIGHEST DECILE

IN HIGHEST DECILE, NOT SIGNIF.

NOT SIGNIF. DIFFERENT FROM U.S.

SIGNIF. LOWER THAN U.S.

Figure 2

Age-adjusted rates of mortality from lung cancer during 1950-75 among white males in rural and urban areas of the Northeast and Southeast

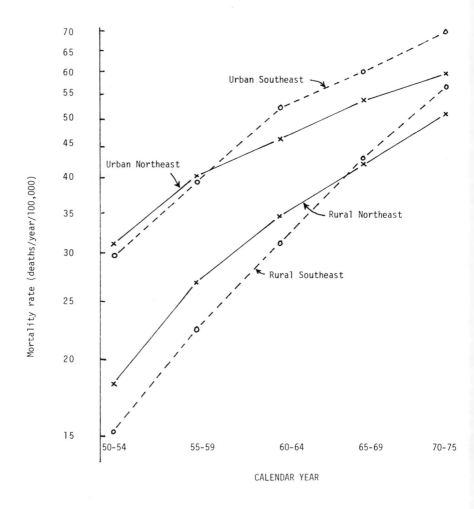

Figure 3

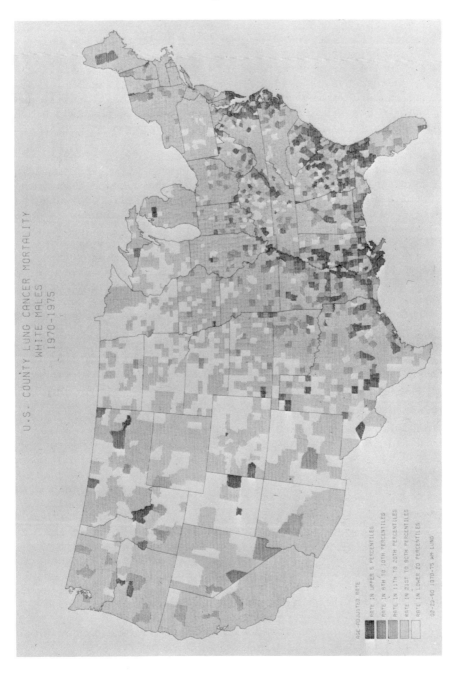

elsewhere and since the reduction in lung cancer risk following cessation of smoking is rather rapid, differential smoking
patterns may also account for some of the changing geographic
patterns for this cancer. Unfortunately, county-level data
on tobacco consumption are not available. It seems unlikely,
however, that smoking patterns explain all the geographic
variation in lung cancer in this country.

In 1969 a cohort study of workers in a copper smelter in
the western U.S. showed an overall 3-fold increased risk of
lung cancer, rising to 8-fold among workers most heavily exposed to arsenic trioxide[7]. When we examined the lung cancer
mortality in all U.S. counties with nonferrous primary
smelters, we found elevated rates in counties with copper,
lead, or zinc smelters (which release inorganic arsenic in
the smelting process) but not in counties with other smelting
and refining operations[8]. The rates tended to be high among
females as well as males. The female excess, along with the
elevated body levels of inorganic arsenic in persons residing
near certain smelters[9], raised the possibility of a community
risk of arsenical air pollution from smelter stacks. This
hypothesis is currently under test by a case-control study of
lung cancer in counties around a particular smelter.

The locations of the smelters were identified from a
large file of public information collected by the Census of
Manufactures (Department of Commerce), which provides the
location and approximate number of employees for all manufacturing plants in the U.S.[10]. Using these data we classified each county as to its relative involvement in each of
18 major industrial classifications. When the lung cancer
rates throughout the U.S. were examined in relation to county-
wide industrial activity, it was found that mortality tended
to be higher in counties with chemical, petroleum, and paper
industries, although the relation to paper production was
limited to the east and south[11]. The elevation in rates in
these counties was small, but was not accounted for by urbani-
zation or other demographic factors, and was primarily in
males. A positive association with transportation manufacturing was also found, particularly with the occupational sub-
category dealing with shipbuilding. There are now few U.S.
counties with major shipyards, but ship construction and
repair comprised the largest manufacturing industry in the
U.S. during World War II, with a peak employment of about 1.7
x 10^6 in late 1943. Among the 49 counties with large shipyards during the war there was a consistent pattern of excess
mortality rates for respiratory cancer during the period
1950-69[12].

To find reasons for the high rates of lung cancer along

the southeast Atlantic coast, we conducted a case-control
study in coastal Georgia, in collaboration with the Center
for Disease Control. Approximately 500 males diagnosed with
lung cancer during 1970-76 (or their next-of-kin) and about
600 controls were interviewed for lifetime histories of
residence, occupation, and smoking. The major finding of
the study was an excess risk associated with employment in
area shipyards during World War II[13]. Two large shipyards in
Brunswick and Savannah began operation in 1942 and by late
1943 together employed about 35,000 persons. Both yards
closed soon after the war. Over 20% of the lung cancer
patients reported work in the shipbuilding industry, almost
all for just a few years during the war. The overall relative risk associated with shipyard employment, adjusted for
smoking and other factors, was 1.6, i.e., a 60% excess risk.
There was a synergistic interaction between this employment
and cigarette smoking, with a substantial risk among workers
who were heavy smokers. Although asbestos seems the likely
agent, exposure data were scanty -- few cases reported
actually handling asbestos as part of their shipyard duties.

We next conducted a similar study in Tidewater, Virginia,
in collaboration with the State Health Department. Respiratory cancer mortality in this coastal area is about as elevated as in Georgia. Shipbuilding has long been a major
source of employment in this region. As in Georgia, an
increased risk of lung cancer was associated with shipyard
employment[14]. The excess risk, adjusted for cigarette
smoking, was on the order of 70%, and was primarily among
those who began employment during World War II or earlier.
As shown in Table 1, there was no appreciable difference in
risk between career employees (who averaged over 25 years
work in the shipbuilding industry) and part-time workers (who
averaged over 25 years work in the shipbuilding industry) and
part-time workers (who averaged less than 5 years, usually
during the war). This suggests that shipyard exposures in
the 1940's, most likely to asbestos, are mainly responsible
for the excess risk of lung cancer in recent years.

The role of asbestos was underscored by the clustering
of mesothelioma that was also seen in the Tidewater area.
Over 70 cases were diagnosed during 1972-78, mostly among
white males. Their incidence of this rare and fatal tumor
exceeded the national average by 4-fold[15]. We interviewed
the next-of-kin of over 90% of the mesothelioma patients and
found that over three-fourths had worked in area shipyards --
almost all beginning prior to 1950. About one-third of the
workers were pipecovers or pipefitters, whose asbestos exposure was probably heavy, but for the remaining workers

exposure to asbestos was indirect or not reported. Mesothelioma did not appear to be increased among the female
population of coastal Virginia. However, among the 5 women
diagnosed with this cancer, 4 were married to shipyard
workers.

TABLE 1

Relative risk of lung cancer, adjusted for cigarette smoking,
associated with shipyard employment, Tidewater, Virginia,1976.

Shipbuilding	Employed Before 1950	Lung Cancer Cases	Controls	Adj Relative Risk
Never employed	–	224	266	1.0
Employed, but not usual industry (non-career)	No	9	11	0.8
	Yes	52	39	1.7*
Usual industry (career)	No	8	9	1.1
	Yes	43	36	1.7*

* P < .05

ORAL CANCER

Interesting sex differences were seen in the maps for
cancer of the mouth and pharynx. Males showed elevated rates
in the northeast, particularly urban areas, consistent with
patterns of smoking and alcohol consumption. However,females
had high rates in the south, in both rural and urban areas.
When the oral cancer rates were correlated with industrial
activities, an association was seen among women in southern
counties with textile manufacturing plants[16]. This seemed
consistent with the reported excess of oral tumors in textile
workers in England, but the correlations in the U.S. may have
been influenced by the heavier use of snuff among textile
workers who are encouraged not to smoke because of the fire
hazard. Indeed the high mortality among southern women cor-
responds to a series of clinical reports of "snuff-dipper's
cancer" in several areas of the South. The role of snuff
use appears to be confirmed by preliminary results for a
case-control study of oral cancer, in collaboration with the
University of North Carolina.

ESOPHAGEAL CANCER

The geographic pattern for esophageal cancer resembles that for oral cancer with a northern excess in men but not women. However, the worldwide variation of esophageal cancer is greater than for any other neoplasm, with extremely high rates in parts of northern China, as reported elsewhere in this volume. The U.S. maps for esophageal cancer also show pockets of elevated mortality, particularly among blacks, whose rates are twice as high as in whites. The rates among blacks are especially elevated in northern cities, yet the highest rates were recorded in a cluster of counties around Charleston, South Carolina[17]. Incidence and mortality rates have been increasing among blacks over time, while remaining nearly constant among whites. Reasons for the racial disparity are not clear, but may be related to differential patterns of tobacco and alcohol consumption, which appear to account for the bulk of this cancer in the U.S.[18]. Esophageal cancer rates among Chinese Americans are also about double those in white Americans, for unknown reasons[5].

We are now completing a case-control study of esophageal cancer among black men in Washington, D.C., where the rates are higher than in any other major metropolitan area. Preliminary findings show an influence of tobacco smoking and nutrient deficiency, but the primary risk factor is alcohol intake. Over one-third of the esophageal cancer patients were reported to consume, on the average, one pint or more of whiskey per day.

BREAST CANCER

Breast cancer is the most common cancer among American women. The incidence is high in Western societies generally and low in Japan and China, with the international differences being most pronounced at postmenopausal ages. Within the U.S. there is a significant north-south gradient, with the greatest differences at older ages, as shown in Figure 4. A correlation study suggested that environmental factors (? dietary) exert their strongest influence upon breast cancer that develops at older ages, while the patterns for younger women point to reproductive and genetic determinants[19].

There have also been interesting age-specific changes in breast cancer mortality over time. Mortality at premenopausal ages has declined in the U.S. from the 1950's to the 1970's, while rates at perimenopausal ages rose and then fell, and rates at postmenopausal ages were steady and then increased[20]. The magnitude of the changes was small, but tended to parallel the changing fertility patterns among American women over time. This association may reflect the protective influence of early age-at-first-birth upon subsequent breast cancer risk.

Figure 4

Breast Cancer Mortality, 1950-69,
Among White Females in Urban Counties in the Northeast
Compared to Rural Counties in the South

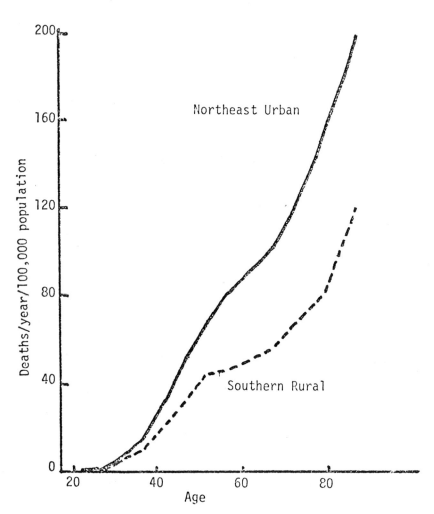

COLORECTAL CANCER

Large bowel cancer is the most common cancer among American men and women combined. Mortality rates for both colon and rectal cancers show a northeastern predominance. Of special interest is the low mortality in those areas of the South such as parts of Florida, Arizona and southern California, that are highly populated with migrants from high-risk areas of the North[21]. Colon cancer rates in the southern retirement areas closely resemble the rates in other urban areas of the south, even at older ages. The patterns raise the possibility that dietary changes associated with moving South have lowered the risk of colon cancer, and perhaps rather rapidly. Field studies are planned in Florida in an effort to identify risk factors, including promoting and inhibiting factors in the diet.

CONCLUSION

In summary, the geographic patterns of cancer in the U.S. are varied and provocative, providing a series of etiologic clues, many of which are now being pursued. As in China, special interest has focused on the unanticipated clusters of counties with elevated mortality for particular cancers. These clusters may be considered as "smoke signals" to environmental hazards that await identification through appropriate epidemiologic and multidisciplinary studies. The geographic studies undertaken by the U.S. and China provide substantial opportunities for bi-national cooperative endeavors. In all likelihood further discoveries will be hastened by closer communication, and by collaborative and parallel efforts designed to unravel the risk factors responsible for the geographic pecularities of cancer in both countries.

REFERENCES

1. Blot WJ, Fraumeni JF Jr, Mason TJ, et al: Developing clues to environmental cancer: a stepwise approach with the use of cancer mortality data. *Environ Health Pers* 32:53-58, 1979.
2. Creech JI and Johnson MN: Angiosarcoma of the liver in the manufacture of polyvinyl chloride. *J Occup Med 16:* 150-151, 1974.
3. Herbst AL, Ulfelder H, and Poskanzer DC: Adenocarcinoma of the vagina: Association of maternal stilbesterol therapy with tumor appearance in young women.

*N Engl J Med 284:*878-881, 1971.
4. Mason TJ and McKay FW: U.S. Cancer Mortality by County: 1950-69. DHEW Publ. No. (NIH) 74-615, U.S. Government Printing Office, Washington, D.C., 1974.
5. Mason TJ, McKay FW, Hoover R, et al: Atlas of Cancer Mortality for U.S. Counties: 1950-69. DHEW Publ. No. (NIH) 75-780, U.S. Government Printing Office, Washington, D.C., 1975.
6. Mason TJ, McKay FW, Hoover R, et al.: Atlas of Cancer Mortality among U.S. Nonwhites: 1950-69. DHEW Publ. No. (NIH) 76-1204, U.S. Government Printing Office, Washington, D.C., 1976.
7. Lee AM and Fraumeni JF Jr: Arsenic and respiratory cancer in man: An occupational study. *J Natl Cancer Inst 42:*1045-1952, 1969.
8. Blot WJ and Fraumeni JF Jr: Arsenical air pollution and lung cancer. *Lancet 2:*142-244, 1975.
9. Milham S and Strong T: Human arsenic exposure in relation to a copper smelter. *Environ Res 7:*176-182,1974.
10. U.S. Department of Commerce: Census of Manufactures 1963. Washington, D.C.: USGPO, 1966.
11. Blot WJ and Fraumeni JF Jr: Geographic patterns of lung cancer in the United States: Industrial correlations. *Am J Epidemiol 103:*539-550, 1976.
12. Blot WJ, Stone BJ, Fraumeni JF Jr, et al: Cancer mortality in U.S. counties with shipyard industries during World War II. *Environ Res 18:*281-290, 1979.
13. Blot WJ, Harrington JM, Toledo A, et al: Lung cancer after employment in shipyards during World War II. *N Eng J Med 299:*620-624, 1978.
14. Blot WJ, Morris LE, Stroube R, et al: Lung and laryngeal cancers in relation to shipyard employment in coastal Virginia. *J Natl Cancer Inst.,* in press.
15. Tagnon I, Blot WJ, Stroube R, et al: Shipbuilding associated mesothelioma in coastal Virginia. *Cancer Res,* in press.
16. Blot WJ and Fraumeni JF Jr: Geographic patterns of oral cancer in the United States: Etiologic implications. *J Chron Dis 30:*745-757, 1977.
17. Fraumeni JF Jr and Blot WJ: Geographic variation in esophageal cancer mortality in the United States. *J Chron Dis 30:*759-767, 1977.
18. Rothman KJ: Alcohol. In Persons at High Risk of Cancer: An Approach to Cancer Etiology and Control. JF Fraumeni, Jr (Ed.), Academic Press, New York, pp. 135-150, 1975.

19. Blot WJ, Fraumeni JF Jr, and Stone BJ: Geographic patterns of breast cancer in the United States. *J Natl Cancer Inst* 59:1407-1411, 1977.

20. Blot WJ: Changing patterns of breast cancer among American women. *Amer J Public Health,* in press.

21. Ziegler R, Blot WJ, Hoover R, et al: Nutritional factors in the low risk of colon cancer in southern retirement areas: a study protocol. *Cancer Res,* in press.

CANCER EPIDEMIOLOGY IN CHINA:
TWO YEARS OF PROGRESS

ROBERT W. MILLER, M.D.
Chief, Clinical Epidemiology Branch
National Cancer Institute

In September 1977, a U.S. Cancer Delegation visited
Canton, a nearby commune, Shanghai, Soochow, Linhsien and
Peking. The trip, sponsored by the Committee for Scholarly
Communications (National Academy of Sciences) with the
Peoples' Republic of China, lasted 22 days. The group had
12 members: 10 physicians, a geographer and a staff member
of the CSCPRC. Although the 10 physicians represented about
25 specialties, they felt at the beginning as if they were
the proverbial blind men examining different parts of an
elephant. By the end of the trip, however, a tremendous
amount of information had been obtained, as exemplified in
the delegation's report, Cancer in China[1].

I made a return trip to Peking and Shanghai two years
later, in November 1979, as a member of a 7-person group
convened by the (U.S.) National Cancer Institute. The ob-
jective was to initiate the U.S.-PRC binational agreement
for scientific exchanges in oncology.

Substantial progress had been made by the Chinese in
their research, especially as it related to epidemiology.
Two members of our group, Frederick P. Li, M.D., and his
wife, Elaine L. Shiang, M.D., had been in China for 3 months
on a Senior Scholarship provided by the CSCPRC. Their
experience proved to be immensely valuable to them (2,3,4,5,6),
and they were able to lay the groundwork for our visit.

MAPS OF CANCER MORTALITY

The biggest advance had been in making maps of cancer
mortality by county. In 1977 we had learned of the experimental map-making which showed rates for cancer by site for
the communes in Kiangsu Province. We were told that data
were being collected in 6 other provinces. It came as a
surprise in 1979 to learn that at the time of our visit 2
years earlier 600,000 health workers had already collected
information for the 3-year interval 1973-75 on causes of
death throughout China. This study, carried out during the

Great Proletariat Cultural Revolution, involved visiting
more than 90% of the households throughout China to determine
who had died during that interval. When cancer was reported,
documentation was sought. The study revealed that about
700,000 deaths per year were due to cancer. The 2.1 million
cancer deaths in the 3 years were the basis for studying
cancer mortality by county. The results showed a variety of
high-rate areas that had, in effect, epidemics of specific
forms of cancer[2].

Six areas with epidemics of esophageal cancer were
identified whereas only one, Linhsien, had previously been
known. The borders of the epidemic for liver cancer along
the southeastern coast were now clearly defined, and attributed at least in part to hepatitis B in this area. In
southern-most China an inland aggregate of high-rate counties
for liver cancer was thought to be due to aflatoxin contami-
nation of food. In southern China boundaries were also
clearly defined for nasopharyngeal cancer. High-rate
counties, apart from the main aggregate, had been populated
by Cantonese who migrated there several generations ago.
This observation adds to the evidence that genetic predis-
position is a factor in susceptibility to the effects of
Epstein-Barr virus, a microbe believed to be important in
the genesis of this neoplasm.

At the mouth of the Yangtze River Schistosoma japonicum
is prevalent, and the maps show high rates of cancer of the
rectum in this area, adding to the previously sparse evidence
that the parasite is involved in the development of this
neoplasm.

Cancer of the penis and of the uterine cervix in husbands
and wives living in Western countries have raised a question
about the connubial transmission of the responsible agent.
The Chinese maps show high rates for cancer of the penis
inside the larger high-rate area for cancer of the uterine
cervix in central China. Consequently, we now have geographic
evidence to support the concept that a common factor is
involved in the genesis of both cancers.

ETHNIC COMPARISONS

During the celebration of National Day on October 1,1977
we had seen national minority groups performing in the parks,
but it had not occurred to us that they might have dissimilar
mortality rates from cancers of various sites. The national
collection of mortality data shows that the Kazak people
have very high rates of cancer mortality in general, and of
esophageal carcinoma in particular. They live side by side

with another national minority group, the Uighurs, who have
low rates of cancer mortality. Further study may reveal
important factors to account for these differences.

THE SHANGHAI TUMOR REGISTRY

In 1977 our Delegation was greatly excited by the discovery that Shanghai had a tumor registry for the entire
city and that data had been analyzed for the year 1975, just
in time for us to hear about it. Data were available for
incidence and mortality in Shanghai since the early 1960s,
but they could not be analyzed during the Cultural Revolution.
By 1979, all these data had been tabulated, and important
new information about cancer by cell type is now available.
Examples include the observation that cancer of the prostate
is rare, as is Ewing's sarcoma of bone[3], whereas stomach
cancer is the most frequent form of neoplasia. One can now
compare incidence in Shanghai with that for Chinese-Americans
and other ethnic groups in the United States.

CANCERS IN DOMESTIC ANIMALS

In 1974 the world learned of gullet cancers in chickens
in Linhsien while at the same time it learned of an epidemic
of human esophageal cancer there[7]. This information came
from a speech made by a Chinese scientist at the International
Cancer Congress in Florence, Italy. During our trip in 1977
we heard about an incredible experiment of nature. To make
room for a reservoir, a commune of 50,000 people was moved
from an area with a high rate of esophageal cancer to a low-
rate area more than 300 miles away. They left their chickens
behind, bought new ones from the cancer-free flocks of their
new neighbors, and beginning 2 years later, these chickens
developed gullet cancers[8]. This remarkable observation indicated that something the migrants carried with them was
responsible. We suspected the formula for Linhsien pickles,
scraps of which were fed to the chickens. In 1977 we were
given samples of these pickles and had them tested in the
Ames system. The results were positive, indicating the
presence of a mutagen that was presumably also a carcinogen.
Lack of diplomatic relations handicapped us in procuring
further samples for the isolation of the mutagen so it could
be identified and tested for carcinogenicity.
     In Canton we heard about a cluster of nasal and naso-
pharyngeal carcinomas in pigs in the area where nasopharyngeal carcinoma is epidemic in man[1]. We were much impressed
with this unpublished finding. The Chinese were more

tentative about it, for they separated the tumors etiologi-
cally on a basis of a very small distance in their anatomic
location; i.e., nasal vs. nasopharyngeal. In 1979 the
Chinese seemed to see much greater potential in the parallel
occurrence than they had 2 years earlier.

In Shanghai we had heard about 2 ducks with hepatocellular carcinoma in the same area that man suffers excess-
ively from this tumor[1]. Neither we nor the Chinese made
much of this concurrence then, but now hepatitis B has been
found to play a role in the duck tumors and is thought to do
the same in the human cancer[9].

Three domestic animal models for human disease provide
the Chinese and the world with a marvelous opportunity for
evaluating factors involved in species that can be studied
experimentally and which have much shorter latent periods for
these cancers. Intervention that protects against the
carcinogenic agent(s) can thus first be recognized in the
domestic animal models and can presage the end of the human
epidemic.

PERCEPTIONS OR MISPERCEPTIONS OF CHINA

In two years the Chinese have virogously moved ahead in
epidemiology under the leadership of Dr. Li Bing. They have
been quick to adopt methods appropriate to their needs in
map-making, cytogenetics, the establishment of a cancer
journal, the issuance of an informative annual report for
the Institute of Cancer Research in Peking, and a hardbound
collection of the staff's publications during the difficult
years, 1958-78. Authorship by name is replacing authorship
by Committee, and individual responsibility for specific
programs is now clearly apparent through the printed word.

So many foreign scientists have visited China that the
novelty must have worn off. We were received, however, with
the same cordiality as before, and the exchange of information
was open.

Tourism is flourishing and the visitors have had their
effect on Chinese fashions. Drab blues, greys and occasional
browns are now punctuated by brightly colored outerwear.
Pigtails are giving way to a variety of contemporary hairdos.
Free markets for farmers are now seen in the cities. Bill-
boards are no longer exclusively for political slogans. They
now contain some advertising -- at least for motion pictures.
Staring crowds in the streets no longer follow foreigners.
Clapping by patients, factory-workers and others -- a sign of
joy upon arrival of visitors, was heard only once during this
trip. Chinese currency has risen in value against the U.S.

dollar -- about 30% in two years. Peking's main streets
now have special lanes for the teeming bicycles, but auto-
mobile horns honk as relentlessly as ever.

REFERENCES

1. Kaplan, H.S. and Tsuchitani, P.J. (eds.): *Cancer in
   China*. Alan R. Liss, Inc., New York, 235 pp., 1978.
2. Li, F.P. and Shiang, E.L.: Cancer mortality in China.
   J. Natl. Cancer Inst. 65:217-221, 1980.
3. Li, F.P., Jin, F., Tu, C-t. and Gao, Y-t.: Incidence of
   childhood leukemia in Shanghai. *Int. J. Cancer 25*:
   701-703, 1980.
4. Li, F.P., Tu, J-T., Liu, F-S. and Shiang, E.L.: Rarity
   of Ewing's sarcoma in China. *Lancet 1*:1255, 1980.
5. Li, F.P. and Shiang, E.L.: Acupuncture and hepatitis B
   infection. *J. Amer. Med. Assn. 243*:1423, 1980.
6. Li, F.P. and.Shiang, E.L.: Screening for oesophageal
   cancer in 62,000 Chinese. *Lancet 2*:804, 179.
7. Miller, R.W.: Letter: High esophageal cancer rates in
   humans and chickens in North China. *J. Natl. Cancer
   Inst. 54*:535, 1975.
8. Institute for Cancer Research, Chinese Academy of
   Medical Sciences, Cancer Hospital of Hubei Province:
   Epidemiology and pathology of pharyngoesophageal cancers
   in domestic fowls from Henan migrant communities and
   native inhabitants in Zhongxian County, Hubei Province.
   Acta Zool. Sin. 22:314-318, 1976.
9. Blumberg, B.: Personal communication.

Cancer Biology: Causation and Diagnosis

A VIRUS-RELATED PROTEIN IN HUMAN BREAST CANCER

S. SPIEGELMAN,* R. MESA-TEJADA,*+ T. OHNO,*
M. RAMANARAYANAN,* R. NAYAK,* J. BAUSCH,*
C. FENOGLIO,∞ AND I. KEYDAR∞

*Institute of Cancer Research and
+Department of Pathology
College of Physicians and Surgeons
Columbia University, New York, N.Y.

∞Faculty of Life Sciences
Department of Microbiology
Tel Aviv University, Ramat Aviv, Israel

INTRODUCTION

Initial Goals

Ten years ago we initiated an effort to see whether the
concepts and methodologies of molecular biology could generate
information relevant to the control or to the treatment of
cancer in man. It is important to emphasize that we did not
regard this attempt as simply another excercise in molecular
biology. Neither were the experiments designed to prove that
viruses are the cause of human cancer either in general or in
particular. Unfortunately, it is not likely that cancer is
one puzzle with a unique solution. It is more probably a
collection of problems resolvable by a set of compatible
alternatives. We have repeatedly pointed out (31-33)) that
the heritable conversion of a normal into a malignant cell can
be explained by any one of the following: a) somatic mutations (induced by chemicals or radiation); b) chromosomal
imbalance; c) chromosomal rearrangements; d) viral transfor-
mations, and e) self-reinforcing epigenetic events. These
are not a set of mutually exclusive alternatives. Providing
support for one of these mechanisms in a particular instance

This research was supported by the National Cancer Institute,
Contract NO1 CP 7-1016 and Grant No. CA-23767.

does not disprove the validity of the others. Any one of
them could be causative in other tumors, in the same tumor in
other hosts, or even in the same tumor in the same host under
different circumstances. If an incontestable demonstration
has been achieved of one of these mechanisms, the strongest
statement one can logically make, may be phrased as follows:
none of the others can be the sole cause of cancer.

<u>Viruses</u> <u>and</u> <u>Human</u> <u>Cancer</u>

We decided to explore the validity of the viral transformation mechanism because of the following two facts:
1) it was a testable hypothesis by molecular hybridization, a
technology with which we were familiar, and 2) the accumulated
information in similar animal diseases supported the existence
of this mechanism in well-documented experiments. We made the
credible assumption that human biology would not be so unique
as to make the animal studies completely irrelevant to the
human disease. On the contrary, it seemed plausible to enter-
tain the working hypothesis that at least some human neoplasias would have a biological basis similar to that observed
in comparable animal models.

Our initial investigations evolved through a number of
stages that are conveniently identified by the questions that
we posed for experimental resolution, and they may be briefly
listed as follows:

1. Do human neoplasias contain RNA molecules possessing
detectable homology to the RNA of tumor viruses known to cause
similar cancers in animal systems?

2. If a positive outcome is obtained, are the RNA molecules identified in the tumors associated with a reverse
transcriptase?

3. If such RNA reverse transcriptase complexes exist in
human tumors, are they encapsulated in particles possessing
the density and size characteristic of RNA tumor viruses?

The availability of the leukemia and mammary tumor systems of the mouse provided us with the viral agents required
to synthesize the radioactive DNA probes used to search for
and to find the corresponding sequences in the particulate
fractions of the corresponding human neoplasias. Thus,
sequences homologous to the RNA of the mouse mammary tumor
were found (1,34) in human breast cancer and, correspondingly,
sequences homologous to some found in the RNA of the Rauscher
leukemia virus were detected in RNA prepared from human mesenchymal tumors (10,11,17). Positive answers to the second and
third questions were obtained via the design of the simultaneous detection test (30). This assay permits the detection

of oncornavirus-like particles by virtue of the fact that they contain the 70S (or 35S) template and the reverse transcriptase (required for synthesis of cDNA) complexed to the RNA template. In these same experiments it was possible to establish that the particles being detected possessed these key diagnostic features as well as the density and size characteristic of the oncornaviruses.

The Generality of Particles in Human Cancers

The invention and perfection of the simultaneous detection test represented an important advance permitting us to bypass the restriction of being confined to those human diseases for which there were comparable animal models with known viral agents. It thus became possible to extend our investigations beyond breast cancer and the mesenchymal tumors to other clinically important human neoplasias. With the aid of this methodology, we, and others, were able to establish that a wide variety of human tumors did indeed contain particles having the physical and biochemical criteria diagnostic of oncornavirus-like particles. The human neoplasias examined included a variety of cancers of the nasopharynx, stomach, colon, lung, brain, ovary, and skin (2,3,7,8,9,12).

Having found the human particles, the question was what to do with them. One would of course like to perform experiments which would test their possible etiologic role. An obvious approach to produce more particles and study their biology was the use of nude mice as a host for either the particles or the cells of the human tumors carrying them. However, we quickly ran into a not-unexpected problem in which apparent tumor material recovered was found to be loaded with murine oncornaviruses. It became clear that this attempt to gain etiologic information and provide a source of human particles was not likely to succeed. The possibility of finding some other susceptible animal was equally bleak. Recall that we have known of the existence of the murine mammary tumor virus for more than forty years, and no one has yet produced a mammary tumor with this virus in any other organism but the mouse. Under these circumstances, it seemed to us that it was the better part of prudence to set aside the question of etiology in favor of a more modest and attainable goal.

The Diagnostic Potential of the Tumor-associated Particles

The data we had amassed thus far on the particles in human tumors could be equally well explained by either one of the following two alternatives; a) The particles cause

the tumors in which they are found; or, b) the tumors cause
the particles. However, whether they be cause or consequence,
the presence of these particles might be exploitable as a
diagnostic signal.

One particularly impressive feature we were repeatedly
able to confirm influenced the direction of our efforts in this
next phase of our investigation. We found that at least a
portion of the sequences in the particles associated with each
tumor site appeared to be unique. Thus, crosshybridization
distinguished the sequences of particles of stomach cancers
from those found in other types of tumors (e.g. colon, lung,
breast, etc.). Even the three tumors of the skin (i.e., basel
cell carcinoma, squamous cell carcinoma, and melanoma) were
found to contain particle sequences that could be differentiated from one another by crosshybridization tests. Sequence
diversity amongst particles from different types of tumors in
the same animal is not a completely new phenomenon. It was
already known to be true for the mouse. Sequences found in
the particles of sarcomas can be distinguished from those
present in leukemias or lymphomas. Those found in mammary
cancer particles are completely unique and do not crosshybri-
dize detectably with any of the particle RNAs found in the
mesenchymal tumors. This kind of individuality appears to be
a general phenomenon with respect to all the particles we have
thus far characterized from the human tumors. The specificity of the sequences found in these particles would appear to
differ not only with respect to the organ of origin, but even
more interestingly, they are histogenically specific.

These results suggested the possibility of developing a
novel pathway for tumor detection. One might perhaps have
imagined that these sequence differences could be directly
employed for this purpose. However, from the outset, it was
evident that the nucleic acid hybridization technology, which
we had developed to provide information on the molecular basis
of the cancer cell, was not likely to be useful in a clinical
setting. The hybridization procedure is too sophisticated,
too tedious and far too expensive to be introduced as a routine procedure in the clinical pathology laboratory.

It was clear to us that we had to find some way of trans-
lating the sequence differences of the tumor particle nucleic
acid to parameters which were amenable to measurements by procedures more commonly employed in the clinical pathology
laboratory. One attractive approach would depend upon the
plausible expectation that the RNA sequence differences observed would be reflected in proteins that might be distin-
guishable antigenically. Were this in fact realized, one
could immediately hope to employ the sensitive and less

restrictive armamentarium of immunology. These procedures
are not only well developed, but they are in routine use in
clinical laboratories.

At this point, we decided to narrow the scope of our
investigations because of a number of factors. Since we had
excellent animal models, we could have embarked on a search
for tumor-specific antigens in either the mesenchymal tumors
or in breast cancer. However, we opted for the latter because
compared to the leukemias, lymphomas and sarcomas, breast
cancer represented a quantitatively more significant problem
in clinical oncology. Further, and perhaps more critically,
was the recognition that in the case of the leukemias, clinicians did have available excellent systemic indicators of the
disease status via examination of peripheral blood cells or
bone marrow aspirates. The situation is much more difficult
in breast cancers and other solid tumors. Here systemic indicators are rare and the problem of both diagnosis and monitoring the disease status during therapy remains largely un-
resolved. There was little doubt that reliable information in
this area could have profound effects on the efficacy of even
the existing treatment modalities of breast cancer. One need
but point to the dramatic effect on the success rate in the
treatment of choriocarcinoma that followed from the discovery
of the indicator hormone, βHCG, in the urine of women with
this tumor.

The search for tumor-specific antigens and their possible
use as diagnostic and monitoring signals is hardly a new idea.
Whatever novelty exists in the approach that we describe here,
lies in the acceptance of the working assumption that a viral-
related protein is a likely candidate for a tumor-specific
antigen. As will be seen, the disocovery of a tumor-specific
antigen in the case of human breast cancer was certainly cata-
lyzed, if not made possible, by this working assumption. In
any case, the animal model provided the reagents which in
fact made the discovery possible.

Before we could explore this pathway of developing a
specific diagnostic and monitoring device, the following two
questions had to be answered: Can particle-related proteins
be detected in the plasma of tumor-bearing individuals? If
present in the plasma, are they useful diagnostic and prognos-
tic signals of the disease status?

Testing the Diagnostic Utility of Particle Proteins with the Murine Mammary Model

To explore the feasibility of this approach, we naturally
chose the murine mammary tumor model. In experiments which study

the value of various MMTV proteins as signals, we identified
gp52 (a glycoprotein with a molecular weight of 52,000 dal-
tons) as the most useful. We developed a radioimmune assay
(26) and established (27) that the circulating blood contains
levels of gp52 which clearly identify tumor-bearing animals.
Metastatic and primary mammary tumors in mice have been detected with complete certainty by increased plasma levels with
gp52. It was subsequently (28) shown that surgical excision
of the tumor is invariably followed within nine days with a
sharp (10-100 fold) decrease of the plasma gp52 levels. Further, the postsurgical behavior of the plasma gp52 is diag-
nostically and prognostically informative as indicated by the
following features: a) all tumor regrowths were correctly
diagnosed by increases in gp52 levels and some were detected
before they were found by palpation; b) relapses were accom-
panied by continued increases in plasma gp52 concentrations
in rates that usually matched the speed of tumor development;
c) the only animals that remained tumor-free at the termina-
tion of the experiment were those that maintained their gp52
levels at or below 15 ng/ml; d) the probability of an
individual's relapsing within a two-week period is much higher
if the gp52 level is above the mean and is almost certain if
it is higher than two standard deviations above the mean.

The same signal was extremely successful in identifying
predictive adjuvant chemotherapeutic modalities which were
successful in suppressing relapse following surgery. Success
was always signaled by striking suppression in the rise of
the gp52 in the plasma. These results were so remarkable that
they stimulated our hope that similar systemic tests might
ultimately be developed for a viral-related protein in the
case of human disease. Any attempt at an extension of this
sort must begin by answering the following questions: a) what
kind of antigen should be sought in the human disease?;
b) where and how should one initially look for it?

Before embarking on a blind quest for an antigen specific
for the human tumor, it would be prudent to take advantage of
the clues supplied by the information gained from our previous
studies of the human disease and its murine counterpart. The
fact that some homology had been shown between the RNAs of the
human tumors and of the murine tumor particles suggested that
an antigenic relation might conceivably exist between one or
another of the proteins of these particles. The plausibility
of this expectation is supported by serological investigations
with sera from breast cancer patients. Antibodies have been
identified which interact with MMTV components (5,6,13,23,24).
Recently (4), migration inhibition studies of leukocytes from
breast cancer patients have provided evidence of crossreac-

tivity with the gp52 of MMTV. Crossreactive components have
also been detected in MCF-7, an established human breast carcinoma cell line (36).

In considering the question of where and how to look for
such antigens, it is important to recognize certain logistical quantitative limitations in transferring technologies
from mice to humans. Thus, the temptation to set up radioimmune assays for crossreacting proteins in human plasma is
likely to meet with disappointment due to the thousand-fold
blood volume difference between mice and humans. Even if, on
a gram basis, a human tumor is every bit as effective as a
mouse tumor in producing plasma antigens, one would still have
to cope with the fact that the signal would be diluted a
thousand-fold in the human as compared with the mouse. Since
in the mouse we are dealing with levels of about 1000 ng/ml in
heavily-tumored mice, this would mean that for humans with a
comparable tumor level we would be at the level of 1 ng/ml.
For this and other reasons, we decided to focus on the tumor
itself as the most plausible site to initiate the search.

Immunohistochemical Localization of MMTV in Mouse Mammary Tumors

We again turned to the murine model to help develop a
convenient, reliable, and sensitive microscopic method for
identifying viral-related proteins in the cells. Most previous investigators have used immunofluorescence for the
localization of MMTV proteins in mouse mammary tumor tissues
(22). The limitations and disadvantages inherent in the routine use of this particular technique led us to explore the
immunoperoxidase method as more suitable to our immediate
purpose and future needs.

Aside from its applicability to immunoelectromicroscopy,
the immunoperoxidase staining procedure has three major advan-
tages that make it an exceedingly attractive method for antigen localization with conventional bright field microscopy
(18). Briefly, these are as follows: 1) The positive reaction appears as a brown precipitate that, in combination with
an appropriate counterstain, provides sufficient histologic
detail to permit precise histological identification and cytological localization. 2) The preparations do not fade and
thus can be filed as permanent records for future comparison.
3) Paraffin sections can be used if the antigenic determinants of the substance being localized withstand the routine
fixation and embedding procedures required.

In view of our ultimate goal to transfer this technology
to human material, the possibility of using paraffin sections
was particularly attractive. We therefore carried out a com-

parison of the immunohistochemical localization of MMTV antigens in parallel paraffin and frozen sections cut from the
same tumor using the indirect immunoperoxidase method and
rabbit anti-MMTV immunoglobulin IgG. In agreement with previous experience (18) with other antigens, we found that
localization of MMTV antigens in the mammary tumor is visua-
lized with greater precision and sensitivity in the paraffin
sections than in frozen sections (14). This may be attributed
to the superior fixation and preservation of cytologic integ-
rity that results from paraffin embedding as compared to frozen sections in which diffusion of antigen and cellular destruction occur frequently.

We begin with a few representative examples of mouse mammary tumor sections stained with rabbit antibody against mouse
mammary tumor virus (α-MMTV) and monospecific antibody (α-gp52)
raised against the 52,000 dalton glycoprotein, gp52. Included
also are specificity tests achieved by absorptions of the antibodies with relevant antigens, an examination which will be
further detailed when we consider the reactions observed with
human materials.

Figures 1a and 1e show positive reactions obtained with
rabbit antibody (IgG) against whole MMTV (α-MMTV) and with IgG
against purified gp52 (α-gp52) on primary tumors. The princi-
pal difference is in the amount of staining, the intensity
usually being greater when the α-MMTV reagent is used.

The specificity of the immunohistochemical reaction was
examined by selective absorption experiments, and these are
also illustrated in Figure 1. While absorption of α-MMTV completely removes the staining reaction (Figure 1b) only partial
elimination is seen if the absorption of α-MMTV is carried out
with purified gp52 as seen in Figure 1c. On the other hand,
absorptions of the monospecific α-gp52 with gp52 completely
abolishes the reaction as shown in Figure 1f. It is apparent
that the α-MMTV is detecting antigens other than gp52 in these
mouse tumors, a result in accordance with its known polyspeci-
fic nature. Comparisons of Figures 1a and 1d show that absorptions of the α-MMTV with an unrelated virus (e.g. Rauscher
leukemia virus) does not lead to any alteration in the staining reaction.

A few words may be noted about the histological pattern
of the staining. The tumors were all adenocarcinomas and displayed primarily cytoplasmic staining which differed in detail
according to the histologic differentiation in the tumor.
Thus, in well-differentiated areas where the tumor cells
approximate normal or lactating mammary gland structures, the
stain is finely granular located primarily above the nucleus,
increasing in intensity toward the apical borders of the cells

Figure 1

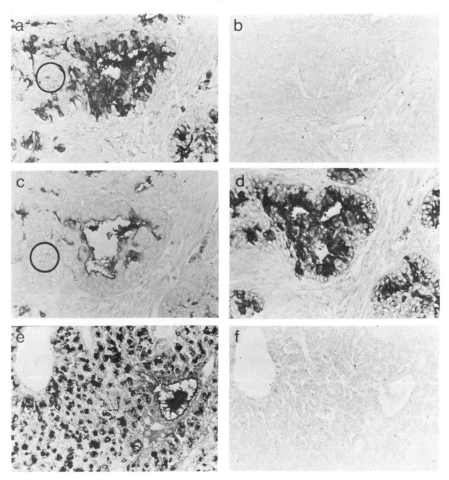

Figure 1. (a-d) Immunoperoxidase stain of same microscopic
field in serial sections of CD8Fl mammary adenocarcinoma,
using as primary antibody α-MMTV (a) and α-MMTV absorbed with
MMTV (b), gp52 (c), and RLV (d), respectively. Antigen localization is greater in cells lining tumor-gland lumina,
whereas more peripheral cells and cell clusters (circled
areas) stain weakly or not at all. Note complete absence of
reaction product in (b) mostly luminal border stain in (c), and
essentially no difference between (a) and (d). (e-f) Immunoperoxidase stain of Paris RIII mammary adenocarcinoma with
α-gp52.(f) Reaction product in (e) is coarsely granular and
unevenly distributed except in tumor gland at right, where

that outline the gland lumen (Figure 1a). Secretions frequently found within these lumina are always darkly stained.
On the other hand, in areas of poor histologic differentiation
where the tumor cells have grown in clusters or sheets, the
intracellular staining consists primarily of coarse irregular
granules unevenly distributed around the nucleus (Figure 1e).
       A certain degree of variability in the amount of staining
as to the number of cells and the amount of staining per cell
was noted within an individual tumor and among the various
tumors tested, a situation, as will be seen below, also seen
with human material. Thus, in addition to quantitative
differences in staining intensity, one may also observe occasional cells or cell clusters that do not stain at all (see
circled areas of Figures 1a and c). In agreement with investigations using immunofluorescence (37), the staining pattern
varies according to the degree of histologic differentiation
of the tumor. In areas of poor differentiation, the staining
is sparse to absent. Wherever the tumor forms glands, a
greater amount of reaction product is noted in the cells and
in the secretions within these glands. A recent (29) investigation reports similar findings with the immunoperoxidase
procedure.
       Before concluding the discussion of the mouse tumors, it
should be emphasized that we deliberately chose highly infected mouse strains to optimize the chances of observing positive reactions and perfecting our method of localizing the
MMTV antigens. Nevertheless, even in these mouse mammary
tumors, MMTV antigens could not be detected in numerous
cells that were obviously malignant. This cellular heterogeneity is frequently observed also in human tumors with respect to other tumor-associated antigens (35).

Immunological Detection in Human Breast Carcinomas

       The technology worked out with the murine mammary tumors
was applied to human material using a variety of poly and
monospecific antisera raised against various protein components of the mouse mammary tumor virus. We quickly detected
evidence for the presence of an antigen in human breast cancer which showed crossreactivity with the gp52 of MMTV.
       In the series to be described, serial sections for
immunohistochemical staining were cut from paraffin blocks of
tissues used for diagnostic purposes selected from the files
of the Divisions of Surgical and Gynecological Pathology of
distribution is typical of well-differentiated areas. Other
clear areas are vascular spaces. Methylene blue counterstain:
Magnification, 155 X.

the College of Physicians and Surgeons of Columbia University.
Additional breast cancer cases were kindly provided by Dr.
Marvin Rich of the Michigan Cancer Foundation and Dr. Y.
Hirschaut of Memorial Sloan-Kettering Cancer Center. The
former were received in the form of unstained paraffin sections and the latter as fresh tumor tissues to be used primarily for antigen isolation studies and from which small sections were fixed and embedded in paraffin for immunohistochemical staining.

The methods and reagents used on the human tissues were
essentially the same (19,20) as those employed on the mouse
mammary tumor studies (14). It is useful to begin by illus-
trating a positive reaction and its elimination by absorption
of the reacting antisera with relevant antigens. Figure 2a
illustrates an intraductal and invasive type of breast carcinoma and a metastatic tumor in the ovary is shown in
Figure 2c. Both show clear evidence of a positive reaction.
The specificity of the positive reactions was examined by
selective absorptions with a variety of absorbants. Comparison of Figures 2b and 2d with their positive counterparts
(Figures 2a and 2c, respectively) reveals that after absorption with purified gp52, the α-MMTV is unable to evoke a
reaction in the carcinomas. The results of absorptions with
other materials are discussed below.

The pattern of staining is quite well exemplified in
Figures 2a and 2c and may be briefly noted. The reactions
observed are primarily focal, intracellular and cytoplasmic.
The considerable staining variability encountered among
different tumors, and also amongst individual cells within
a given tumor is well illustrated in these two examples.
Note in Figure 2a that only some of the cells in the intraductal lesion are stained whereas most of the surrounding
invasive cells contain reactive product. In instances in
which many sections were cut from the same block, some levels
showed more stained cells than others. In other cases not
all blocks from the same tumor gave a positive reaction. It
is evident that the human material shows the same type of
heterogeneity that we have already encountered in the case
of the mouse mammary tumor.

Malignant Breast Tissues

Up to the present time, a positive staining reaction has
been observed in 212 (47.4%) of 447 randomly selected cases
of human breast carcinoma tested, including those received
from other institutions (Table 1). The results observed in

Figure 2

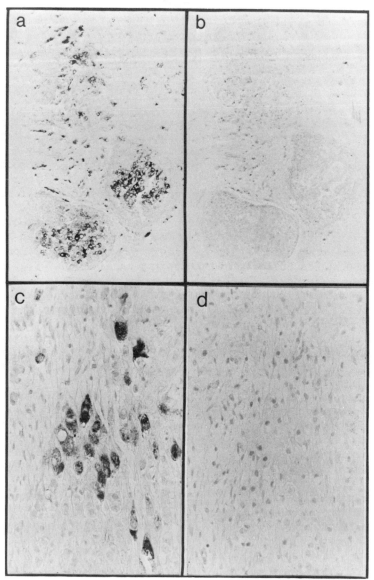

Figure 2. Immunoperoxidase stain of primary and metastatic breast carcinoma with α-MMTV. In the intraductal and invasive tumor (a), some of the cells in the intraductal lesions and most of the invasive cells are stained. Likewise, in the metastatic lesion of the ovary (c), not all of the tumor cells

Table 1

Immunoperoxidase Staining of Carcinoma of the Breast

	Total cases classified as to source		
	Cases	Positive	% Positive
Columbia-Presbyterian	274	133	48.5
Memorial Sloan- Kettering	69	31	44.9
Michigan Cancer Foundation	104	48	46.2
	447	212·	47.4

the Columbia-Presbyterian breast cancer series are subdivided
with respect to histopathologic types in Table 2. It will be
noted that a significantly larger percentage of positive
cases occurs in the mixed intraductal and invasive group
(64.4%), a trend noted in our original report (19) of 131
cases. It appears, therefore, that an invasive carcinoma
associated with an intraductal component is more likely to
contain a crossreacting antigen than either a purely intraductal or purely invasive tumor.

We should now like to illustrate further the features of
the staining reaction in a variety of sections from human
breast cancer material. In this connection, we have chosen
to illustrate both the wide variation in intensities as well
as the high degree of specificity of the reaction. The invasive tumor illustrated in Figure 3a represents the strongest
staining reaction we have yet observed in the human tumor
and compares in intensity with that seen in the mouse mammary
tumor with the same reagents. Note however, that absorption
of the antiserum with purified gp52 (Figure 3b) completely
eliminates even this strong reaction. A dramatic illustration

---

are stained; (b) and (d) are serial sections adjacent to (a)
and (c) in which the reaction has been eliminated by prior
absorption of α-MMTV with gp52. Methylene blue counterstain:
(a); (b) Magnification, 29 X; (c); (d) Magnification, 153 X.

Table 2

Immunoperoxidase Staining of Carcinoma of the Breast

	Histopathologic classification of: Columbia-Presbyterian Cases		
	Cases	Positive	% Positive
Intraductal	25	10	40.0
Intraductal & Invasive	73	47	64.4
Invasive	109	53	48.6
Medullary	18	7	38.9
Metastatic	49	16	32.7
	274	133	48.5

Figure 3

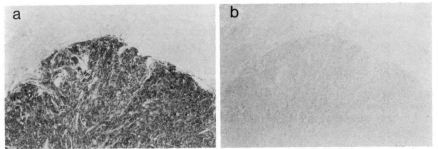

Figure 3. Immunoperoxidase stain of invasive breast carcinoma
with α-MMTV before (a) and after (b) absorption with gp52.
Note in (a), strong reaction in practically all tumor cells
and absence of stain in surrounding connective tissue within
which are morphologically benign ducts and blood vessels.
This strong reaction is not seen in adjacent serial section
(b) treated with gp52-absorbed α-MMTV. Methylene blue counterstain: Magnification, 25 X.

of the exquisite specificity of the reaction is seen in
Figure 4a. Here a positive staining is observed only in the
small focus of invasive carcinoma and no reaction product is
detected in either the surrounding fibrous tissues or in the
neighboring morphologically benign epithelial tissues such as
the adjacent hyperplastic lobules. Again, absorption with
gp52 (Figure 4b) completely eliminates the reaction seen in
the malignant area.

Figure 4

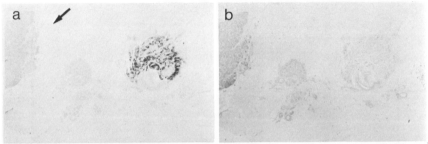

Figure 4. Another field in same section as Figure 3 showing
staining of small focus of invasive carcinoma (a) and lack of
reaction in nearby hyperplastic lobule (arrow) as well as complete elimination of the former reaction after absorption
with gp52 (b). Methylene blue counterstain: Magnification,
25 X.

Figure 5 was chosen to illustrate the sensitivity of the procedure in picking out and identifying the nature of microscopic metastatic lesions. We have here (Figure 5a) a low
power view of an axillary lymph node showing staining in two
microscopic areas. That only one of them contains breast
cancer cells (Figure 5a, large arrow and inset) is demonstrated by its elimination (Figure 5b, large arrow and inset)
after absorption with gp52. The other area (Figure 5a, short
arrow) contains erythrocytes in a small blood vessel and the
staining is due to the presence of endogenous peroxidase or
some other irrelevant material, a reaction which is not eliminated (Figure 5b, short arrow) by absorption with gp52.
The insets of Figures 5a and 5b show that most of the neoplastic cells in the micro tumor stain with α-MMTV and that
this reaction is completely eliminated by absorption with
gp52.
     The reactions seen in Figure 5 and in the ovarian meta-
stases of Figure 2 illustrate how with proper controls, the
immunohistochemical technique can be used to help locate

and identify the origin of microscopic malignant lesions.
Many of these might well be missed or ambiguously diagnosed
by the procedures usually employed.

Figure 5

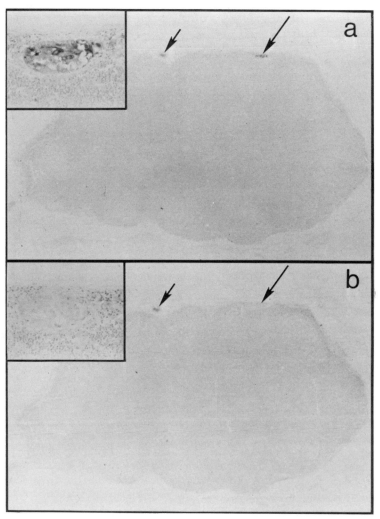

Figure 5. Axillary lymph node from patient with invasive
carcinoma of the breast showing metastatic lesions in margi-
nal sinus (long arrows, insets). Most of the neoplastic
cells stain with anti-gp52 (a); this reaction is eliminated
by absorption with gp52 (b). Note that stain seen in erythrocytes in small blood vessel (short arrows) is unaffected by

In evaluating the results illustrated above, it is important to realize that there is considerable sampling error inherent in our testing procedure and therefore the percentages
given in Tables 1 and 2 represent, at best, minimal values.
This conclusion is based on the following facts: 1) Diagnostic tissue blocks of a given case are usually representative
of, but seldom include, the entire tumor. 2) These studies
were limited to an average of less than three (one, in cases
from other institutions) representative blocks per case, and
as previously noted, there was a considerable variability in
antigen localization among and within sections of positive
cases. 3) In contrast to in vitro methods, where a given
tissue can be analyzed in bulk, our test is limited to 5 μm
sections, which represent only a minute fraction of the entire
tumor (approximately 1/1000 of a 0.5-cm tumor).

Normal and Benign Breast Tissues

We have already seen (e.g., in Figure 4) that normal and
benign tissue in the same section do not show evidence of the
tumor-specific antigen exhibited by a contiguous malignant
area. It is therefore not surprising that we obtained negative results when we examined normal (resting and lactating)
and benign (cystic disease, fibroadenoma, intraductal papil-
loma, and gynecomastia) tissues from 137 patients (Table 3)
it should be noted that 74 of these negatively staining benign
lesions coincided with the presence of positively staining
carcinoma in the same breast and frequently in the same tissue
section.

Apocrine Metaplasia

The only exception to the absence of staining reaction in
non-malignant breast tissue was the focal staining observed in
apocrine metaplasia, one of the microscopic features of cystic
disease. This reaction is shared by the morphologically and
histochemically indistinguishable epithelium of apocrine glands
of the axilla and perineum. However, as will be detailed below, the apocrine reaction differs in specificity from that
observed in the carcinomas.

---

the absorption, indicating endogenous peroxidase activity or
nonspecific reaction. Methylene blue counterstain: Magnification, 12 X. Insets Magnification, 60 X.

Table 3

Immunoperoxidase Staining of Benign and Normal

Breast Tissues

Type	Cases	Associated with breast carcinoma[*]	Positives
Cystic disease[†]	81	60	0
Fibroadenoma	19	4	0
Intraductal papilloma	10	10	0
Gynecomastia	9	0	0
Resting gland (normal)	9	0	0
Lactating gland (normal)	9	0	0
TOTAL	137	74	0

[*] In the same breast.

[†] Excluding foci of apocrine metaplasia.

Malignancies Other than Breast Carcinomas

Table 4 summarizes the results observed in 99 primary carcinomas from other organs and eight cases of cystosarcoma phyllodes. Only one of these 107 tumors, a mucoepidermoid carcinoma of the parotid gland, gave a positive reaction. Two other parotid carcinomas of the same histopathologic type were negative. It is therefore evident that the antigen being detected by the anti-MMTV and anti-gp52 in human breast carcinomas is confined principally to malignant epithelial cells of mammary gland origin.

The Specificity of the Immunoperoxidase Reaction in Human Breast Carcinomas

The tissue specificity of the staining reaction was discussed in the preceding paragraphs and it appears that a positive specific reaction is confined principally to the cytoplasm of breast carcinoma cells. A precise evaluation of the immunologic specificity in immunohistochemical staining reactions demands meticulous specific absorptions of the primary antibodies not only with homologous antigens but also with

Table 4

Immunoperoxidase Staining of Malignancies Other

than Breast Carcinomas

Malignancy	Cases	Positive
Colon	12	0
Stomach	3	0
Pancreas	3	0
Liver	4	0
Lung	9	0
Endometrium	22	0
Ovary	20	0
Prostate	8	0
Kidney	5	0
Urinary bladder	4	0
Skin	2	0
Thyroid gland	4	0
Parotid gland	3	1
Cystosarcoma phyllodes	8	0
TOTAL	107	1

Primary sites of non-breast carcinomas stained with α-MMTV.
Cystosarcoma phyllodes is also listed because it is the most
common noncarcinomatous malignancy of the breast.

---

related antigens that might be responsible for undesirable or
irrelevant crossreactive phenomena. We therefore used
numerous immunoabsorbants for this purpose. Their preparation and the conditions of absorption have been described in
detail elsewhere (21).

The outstanding difference between mouse and human tumors
with respect to antigen localization with anti-MMTV is readily
apparent. In contrast with mouse tumors where only absorptions with whole disrupted MMTV completely eliminated the
staining reaction (see Figures 1a, 1b, 1c), absorption with
gp52 alone was sufficient to obliterate the reaction in positive staining human tumors (Figures 2b, 2d, 3b, 4b). A reaction in human tissues, therefore, was considered positive

only when a) definite staining was seen, and b) the staining
was completely absent in an adjacent serial section stained
with the same antibody preparation previously absorbed with
gp52. We further explored the specificity of the staining
reaction by absorption with the various preparations of MMTV
and gp52 listed in Table 5. The fact that all eliminated the
staining reaction indicates that the species differences previously reported (22) for gp52 of the C3H and RIII strain of
MMTV do not play a role in this reaction. On the other hand,
absorptions with unrelated preparations (Rauscher leukemia
virus, Simian Sarcoma virus, Mason-Pfizer monkey virus, and
Baboon Endogenous virus) and with several possible crossreacting substances, also listed in Table 5, failed to eliminate the staining reaction. Further, the source of gp52
(C3H or RIII), and the host cell of the virus (murine cells or
feline cells), had no influence on the ability to eliminate
the crossreactivity from the antibodies tested.

These absorptions also led us to suspect that the staining observed in the apocrine epithelium differs in specificity
from the reaction observed in the carcinomas, for the
following reasons: 1) Absorption with gp52 blocks only part
of the reaction in the apocrine glands and metaplasia while
completely eliminating the reaction in the carcinomas. If
this absorption is carried out with gp52 that has not previously been extracted with ether, both reactions are completely blocked. 2) Absorption with mucin almost completely
eliminates the reaction of the apocrine epithelium but does
not interfere with the staining of the carcinoma, indicating
that the reaction in the apocrine material is due, at least
in part, to a carbohydrate moiety.

The Role of the Sugar Residues in the Crossreactivity of gp52 with the Human Breast Cancer Antigen

It was of some practical importance to establish whether
the sugar or protein moiety of gp52 was responsible for its
ability to block the immunological crossreaction with the antigen found in human breast cancer cells. Aside from its genetic and etiologic implications, the outcome could materially
influence the nature of our attempts to isolate, to characterize, and to devise assay procedures for the human tumor-
specific antigen.

Sugar-free gp52 was prepared by deglycosylation of
(^{3}H)glucosamine-labeled gp52. The effectiveness of the removal
of the carbohydrate was monitored on the recovered polypeptide
by residual tritiumstaining with periodic acid Schiff (PAS)reac-
tion, and by quantitative assay for carbohydrate by the ferri-

TABLE 5

Absorption Specificity Tests of Immunoperoxidase
Staining of Human Breast Carcinoma with α-MMTV*

Completely Eliminated by:	Not Eliminated by:
MMTV (RIII) from milk	**Viruses**
MMTV (C3H) from MM5T	Rauscher leukemia virus
MMTV (C3H) from CrFeK	Simian sarcoma virus
	Mason-Pfizer monkey
gp52 (RIII) ⎫ Purified by conca-	virus
gp52 (C3H) ⎬ navalin A affinity	Baboon endogenous virus
chromatography	**Human**
	normal plasma
gp52 (RIII) ⎫ Purified by guani-	normal leukocytes
gp52 (C3H) ⎬ dium chloride	collagen
chromatography	actin
	hyaluronic acid
	milk
	normal breast tissue
	Bovine
	mucin
	fetal calf serum
	Sheep erthrocytes

*The absorptions were done by using these agents either in
the soluble or insolubilized form.

cyanide method (16). The data indicate that of the 20 sugar
residues per polypeptide chain originally present in gp52,
less than one third of a residue per chain remained after deglycosylation. Nevertheless, the deglycosylated gp52 was as
effective in removing the immunohistochemical reaction in
human tumors as was absorption with the untreated gp52 (25).
The outcomes of such absorption experiments are exemplfied
in Figure 6 by a uniquely informative tissue sample from a
patient with intraductal and invasive breast carcinoma. We
have here in the same section a nipple duct containing lobu-
lar carcinoma in situ, a nearby normal duct, and another duct
exhibiting apocrine metaplasia. The insets allow one to compare at higher magnifications the staining of malignant cells
(lower right hand corner) and of the apocrine metaplasia
(upper left hand corners). Prior to absorption with gp52
(Figure 6a), the intraductal tumor stains heavily, the apocrine epithelium shows its usual focal granular staining at
the apex and glycocalyx and the normal duct does not stain at
all. After absorption of the α-gp52 with deglycosylated gp52
(Figure 6b), all reaction disappears from the malignant cells
in the duct but the staining of the apocrine metaplasia is
not appreciably decreased. Thus the human malignant antigen
is crossreacting with the polypeptide portion of gp52 whereas
the apocrine antigen is immunologically related to the carbohydrate moiety. This result is in accordance with our
earlier findings (21) that absorption of α-MMTV with mucin
failed to modify the reaction with breast cancer cells, but
markedly suppressed the reactivity with apocrine metaplasia.

Implications and Prospects

The fact that it is the polypeptide, rather than polysaccharide portion of the gp52, that is responsible for the
immunological reactivity with the human breast cancer antigen
adds additional significance to the biological similarities
between the human and murine mammary neoplasias. At the very
least, this outcome indicates that the immunologic relationship between the human breast cancer antigen and gp52 is more
than a chance correspondence of polysaccharide complexes.
     It is of course gratifying to have extended to the pro-
tein level the relation between human breast cancer and MMTV
that was initially discovered (1) in terms of nucleic acid
homology. However, our immediate concern is not with etiological implications of these findings but rather with the
possibility that their extension could generate clinically
useful information. To this end our present efforts are

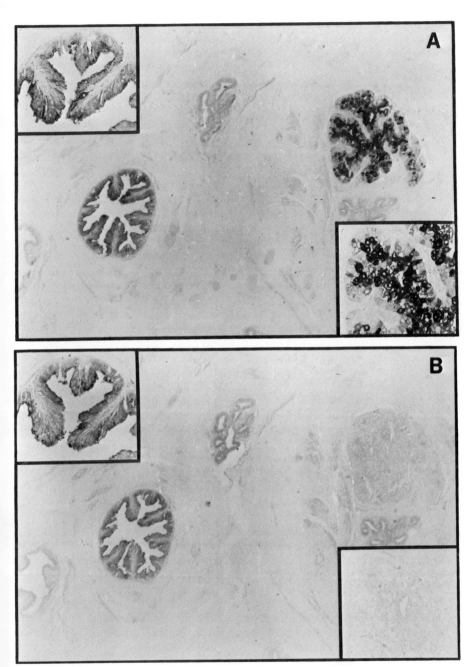

Figure 6. (a) Immunoperoxidase stain with α–MMTV of cross section of nipple duct from a case of intraductal and invasive

focused on the following issues; 1) How widespread is this
antigen in the human population, with particular reference to
frequency and severity of the disease? 2) Can any correlations be drawn between antigen levels in the diseased tissue
and identifiable clinical parameters? 3) What is the nature
of the crossreacting human breast cancer antigen and how is
it related chemically to gp52? 4) Can an assay for the human
antigen be developed which would meet the sensitivity levels
required to detect this antigen in the body fluids of
patients?

Answers to the first two questions are being actively
pursued through collaborative efforts set up with cancer cen-
ters here and in foreign countries, including Germany, Holland, Japan, Tunisia, and Israel. It is already evident that
the breast cancer antigen is globally distributed and that
its level appears to correlate with the frequency and severity
of the disease. We have further noted in our own local population that a significantly greater number of breast cancer
patients with a family history of breast cancer expressed the
gp52 crossreactive antigen when compared to patients with no
such family history.

Complete resolution of the last two questions will require
purification to homogeneity of the human breast cancer antigen.
The logistical feasibility of attaining this goal has been
achieved by the establishment of a cell line (15) from the
pleural effusion of a patient with intraductal and invasive
breast carcinoma. This cell line (T47D) and its clonal derivatives express the gp52-related antigen. The antigen is
shed into the supernatant in a particulate form making its
isolation relatively convenient. We have already identified
and isolated an 80 amino acid polypeptide fragment from gp52
which carries the human-related reactivity and we should soon
be able to do the same for the human antigen.

---

carcinoma of the breast, showing one duct involved by in situ
carcinoma (right) and another with apocrine metaplasia (left).
Inset: details of the above, showing considerable intracellular reaction product in the neoplastic cells and characteristic intracellular granular staining in the apocrine epithelium. (b) Immunoperoxidase stain of adjacent serial section
using anti-MMTV previously absorbed with sugar-free gp52.
Note complete absence of reaction product in the neoplastic
cells, whereas the intensity of the staining reaction in the
apocrine epithelium is essentially the same as in (a). Methylene blue counterstain: Magnification, 38 X. Insets:
Magnification, 94 X.

The availability of the 47D culture will facilitate the production of the monoclonal antibodies via hybridomas which will be needed to develop the heterologous immunoassays that can hope to attain the sensitivities required for the development of a systemic signal for human breast cancer.

REFERENCES

1. Axel, R., J. Schlom, and S. Spiegelman, (1972a).
    Presence in human breast cancer of RNA homologous to
    mouse mammary tumor virus RNA. Nature 235: 32.
2. Axel, R., S.C. Gulati, and S. Spiegelman, (1972b). Par-
    ticles containing RNA-instructed DNA polymerase and
    virus-related RNA in human breast cancers. Proc. Nat.
    Acad. Sci. USA 69: 3133.
3. Balda, B.-R., R. Hehlmann, J.-R. Cho, and S. Spiegelman,
    (1975). Oncornavirus-like particles in human skin
    cancers. Proc. Nat. Acad. Sci. USA 72: 3697.
4. Black, M.M., R.E. Zachrau, A.S. Dion, B. Shore, D.L.
    Fine, H.P. Leis, Jr., and C.J. Williams, (1976). Cellu-
    lar hypersensitivity to gp55 of RIII-murine mammary tu-
    mor virus and gp55-like protein of human breast cancers.
    Cancer Res. 36: 4137.
5. Bowen, J.M., L. Dmochowski, M.F. Miller, E.S. Priori,
    G. Seman, M.L. Dodson, and K. Maruyama, (1976). Implica-
    tions of humoral antibody in mice and humans to breast
    tumor and mouse mammary tumor virus-associated antigens.
    Cancer Res. 36: 759.
6. Charney, J., and D.H. Moore, (1971). Neutralization of
    murine mammary tumor virus by sera of women with breast
    cancer. Nature 229: 627.
7. Chezzi, C., G. Dettori, V. Manzari, A.M. Agliano, and
    A. Sanna, (1976). Simultaneous detection of reverse
    transcriptase and high molecular weight RNA in tissue of
    patients with Hodgkin's disease and patients with leuke-
    mia. Proc. Nat. Acad. Sci. USA 73: 4649.
8. Cuatico, W., J.-R. Cho, and S. Spiegelman, (1973). Par-
    ticles with RNA of high molecular weight and RNA-directed
    DNA polymerase in human brain tumors. Proc. Nat. Acad.
    Sci. USA 70: 2789.
9. Cuatico, W., J.-R. Cho, and S. Spiegelman, (1974). Evi-
    dence of particle-associated RNA-directed DNA polymerase
    and high molecular weight RNA in human gastrointestinal
    and lung malignancies. Proc. Nat. Acad. Sci. USA 71:
    3304.
10. Hehlmann, R., D. Kufe, and S. Spiegelman, (1972). Viral-
    related RNA in Hodgkin's disease and other human lympho-
    mas. Proc. Nat. Acad. Sci. USA 69: 1727.
11. Hehlmann, R., D. Kufe, and S. Spiegelman, (1972). RNA in
    human leukemic cells related to the RNA of a mouse leu-
    kemia virus. Proc. Nat. Acad. Sci. USA 69: 435.
12. Hehlmann, R., B.-R. Balda, and S. Spiegelman, (1978).
    Murine and human melanomas containing a high molecular
    weight RNA associated with an RNA-instructed DNA poly-

merase. Int. J. Dermatol. 17: 114.

13. Holder, W.D., Jr., G.W. Peer, D.P. Bolognesi, and S.A. Wells, Jr.,(1976). Antibody reacting with mouse mammary tumor virus in serum of breast carcinoma patients. Surg. Forum 27: 102.

14. Keydar, I., R. Mesa-Tejada, M. Ramanarayanan, T., Ohno, C. Fenoglio, R. Hu, and S. Spiegelman, (1978). Detection of viral proteins in mouse mammary tumors by immunoperoxidase staining of paraffin sections. Proc. Nat. Acad. Sci. USA 75: 1524.

15. Keydar, I., L. Chen, S. Karby, F.R. Weiss, J. Delarea, M. Radu, S. Chaitcik, and H.J. Brenner, (1979). Establishment and characterization of a cell line of human breast carcinoma origin. Europ. J. Cancer 15: 659.

16. Krystal, G., and A.F. Graham, (1976). A senstitive method for estimating the carbohydrate content of glycoproteins. Anal. Biochem. 70: 336.

17. Kufe, D., W.P. Peters, and S. Spiegelman, (1973). Unique nuclear DNA sequences in the involved tissues of Hodgkin's and Burkitt's lymphomas. Proc. Nat. Acad. Sci. USA 70: 3810.

18. Mesa-Tejada, R., R.R. Pascal, and C.M. Fenoglio, (1977). Immunoperoxidase: A sensitive immunohistochemical technique as a "special stain" in the diagnostic laboratory. Human Pathol. 8: 313.

19. Mesa-Tejada, R., I. Keydar, M. Ramanarayanan, T. Ohno, C. Fenoglio, and S. Spiegelman, (1978a). Detection in human breast carcinomas of an antigen immunologically related to a group-specific antigen of the mouse mammary tumor virus. Proc. Nat. Acad. Sci. USA 75: 1529.

20. Mesa-Tejada, R., I. Keydar, M. Ramanarayanan, T. Ohno, C. Fenoglio, and S. Spiegelman, (1978b). Immunohistochemical detection of a crossreacting virus antigen in mouse mammary tumors and human breast carcinomas. J. Histochem. Cytochem. 26: 532.

21. Mesa-Tejada, R., I. Keydar, M. Ramanarayanan, J. Bausch, and S. Spiegelman, (1979). Immunohistochemical evidence for the presence of RNA virus related components in human breast cancer. Ann. Clin. and Lab. Sci. 9: 202.

22. Moore, D.H., C.A. Long, and A.B. Vaidya. Mammary Tumor Viruses, in: ADVANCES IN CANCER RESEARCH (eds. G. Klein and S. Weinhouse), Vol. 29, p. 347, Academic Press, New York, (1979).

23. Müller, M., and H. Grossman, (1972). An antigen in human breast cancer sera related to the murine mammary tumor virus. Nature 237: 116.

24. Müller, M., C. Kemmer, S. Zotter, H. Grossmann, and B. Michael,(1973). Kreuzreaktion zwischen Brustkrebs und Mastopathie des Menchen sowie murinen Mammkarzinomen: Lokalisation des Antigen im Bereich der A-Partikel des Mammatumorvirus. Arch Geschwulstforch 41: 100.

25. Ohno, T., Mesa-Tejada, R. Keydar, I., Ramanarayanan, M. Bausch, J., and Spiegelman, S.: The human breast carcinoma antigen is immunologically related to the polypeptide of the group-specific glycoprotein of the mouse mammary tumor virus. Proc. Nat. Acad. Sci. USA 76: 2460-2464.

26. Ritzi, E., A. Baldi, and S. Spiegelman, (1976a). The purification of a gs antigen of the murine mammary tumor virus and its quantitation by radioimmunoassay. Virology 75: 188.

27. Ritzi, E., D.S. Martin, R.L. Stolfi, and S. Spiegelman (1976b). Plasma levels of a viral protein as a diagnostic signal for the presence of tumor: The murine mammary tumor model. Proc. Nat. Acad. Sci. USA 73: 4190.

28. Ritzi, E., D.S. Martin, R.L. Stolfi, and S. Spiegelman, (1977). Plasma levels of a viral protein as a diagnostic signal for the prescence of mammary tumor: The effect of tumor removal. J. Exp. Med. 145: 999.

29. St. George, J.A., R.D. Cardiff, L.J.T. Young and L.J. Faulkin, 1979. The immunocytochemical distribution of mouse mammary tumor virus antigens in BALB/cfC3H mammary epithelium. J. Nat. Cancer Inst. 63: 813-820.

30. Schlom, J., and S. Spiegelman(1971). Simultaneous detection of reverse transcriptase and high molecular weight RNA unique to oncogenic RNA viruses. Science 174: 840.

31. Spiegelman, S., (1975). Evidence for viruses in human neoplasias. Haematologica 60: 339.

32. Spiegelman, S., R. Axel, W. Baxt, D. Kufe, and J. Schlom, (1975). The molecular genetics of human cancer and its etiologic implications. Genetics 79: 317.

33. Spiegelman, S., (1976). The Search for Viruses in Human Cancer, in Proceedings of the American Philosophical Society 120: 69.

34. Vaidya, A.B., M.M. Black, A.S. Dion, and D.H. Moore, (1974). Homology between human breast tumour RNA and mouse mammary tumour virus genome. Nature 249: 565.

35. Wolfe, H.J., (1979) Tumor-cell markers: A biologic shell game? New Eng. J.Med. 299: 146.

36. Yang, N.-S., H.D. Soule, and C.M. McGrath,(1977). Expression of murine mammary tumor virus-related antigens in human breast carcinoma (MCF-7) cells. J. Nat. Cancer

Inst. 59: 1357.

37. Zotter, S., M. Müller, and C. Kemmer, (1974). Korrelation zwischen der Produktion reifer Virus-partikel und der histo-morphologischen Differenzierung virus induzierter muriner Mammakarzinome. Arch. Geschwulstforsch 44: 212.

THE NATURE OF CANCER CELLS

RENATO DULBECCO
The Salk Institute

DIFFERENCES BETWEEN CANCER AND NORMAL CELLS

The properties of cancer cells have been studied for
many decades. A great wealth of information shows that cancer
cells differ in very many characteristics from normal cells.
However, the validity of this statement is somewhat weakened
by two facts: 1) the impossibility of studying, in many
cases, the normal cells from which the tumor arose, if they
are present in small numbers; and 2) the quiescent state of
the normal cells, whereas the cancer cells contain a substantial growing function. I shall return to this point later.
The differences between cancer cells and normal cells
affect enzyme activities, types of isozymes[1] antigens[2]
biochemical features of several cell compartments[3,4,5] and
excreted products like hormones, immunoglobulins, collagen,
etc. Very extensive tables of such differences have been
published, but only some of the differences are interesting
in the sense that we can see a rationale for them.
Among these are differences that distinguish metasta-
sizing cells from the cells of the primary tumors. These
have been studied especially with some suitable experimental
systems such as the B16 mouse melanoma or the UV 2237 mouse
fibrosarcoma. The metastatic cells show differences in
surface properties[6] or increased ability to grow in agar[7,8] to
produce plasminogen activator[9] or to break down the collagen
IV of basal membranes[6] These properties show that features
of the cancer cells determine the biology of the neoplasia
and suggest that interactions of the surfaces of the neoplastic cells with those of other cells or with basal
membranes is important in metastasis formation.

ECTOPIC HORMONES AND OTHER PROTEINS

Especially interesting for understanding the nature of
cancer is the production of polypeptide hormones by cancers
developing in organs in which the hormones are not normally
produced (so-called ectopic hormones)[1] The production of
the ectopic hormones together with that of abnormal isozymes
has been studied for determining the relationship of gene
expression in the cancer cells compared to that of normal
cells belonging to a preceding stage of differentiation.
Indeed the expressed genes under the two conditions are
similar in some cases (retrograde expression).[10] But this is not

a general finding; in many instances the genes expressed in
cancer cells are totally unrelated to those expressed in the
cell lineage from which the cancer cells derive. It can be
said that in cancer cells the expression of genes is not
activated in a developmental fashion, but in a rather dis-
orderly way. To make the situation even more complex the
genes expressed in cells of similar cancers can be quite
different, as observed with experimental hepatomas; and
heterogeneity of gene expression is shown by cytological
studies even between cells of the same tumor.[11]

In addition to expression of new genes, cancer cells
usually show loss of expression of other genes. Therefore
the changes of gene expression in cancer are multiple and
varied.

SPECIFIC CANCER CHANGES

In spite of these multiple changes, the dream of
researchers to identify a function strictly characteristic
of cancer cells has not been realized. Restricted antigens,
not shared by other cells or even by similar tumors, are
present in some melanomas or astrocytomas, but they are
isolated instances. Furthermore their restriction has to
pass a more stringent test, as can be provided by extensive
libraries of monoclonal antibodies to defined surface
antigens. A unique surface antigen in a tumor would have a
special meaning. In fact, if the gene specifying the antigen
were cellular, it would have to remain unexpressed throughout
ontogeny and there would be no reason for its evolutionary
persistence. The gene specifying such an antigen would have
a high probability of being viral, or a cellular gene altered
by mutation or recombination.

A few products resulting from retrograde or abnormal
expression, although not exclusive of cancer cells, turn out
to be useful for following the course of the disease. Among
them are carcinoembryonic antigen, α-fetoprotein or a special
isozyme of galactosyl transferase, measured in the blood.
Regular differentiation products can also fulfill this role
if they are regularly produced by the cancer cells (like
chorionic gonadotropin with choriocarcinoma). The potential
of these various approaches for defining and identifying
cancers will become evident after the present efforts of many
laboratories will have generated a broad library of monoclonal
antibodies to surface antigens of normal and neoplastic cells.
Then it will be possible to establish in an unambiguous way
the association of specific, well-defined surface antigens
and cancer cells of various types.

CANCER MARKERS AS REPLICATION MARKERS

Recent observations show that some of the many differences of gene expression observed in cancer cells are also observed in replicating normal cells; these differences may thus be attributed to the presence of a sizeable proportion of replicating cells in any cancer. In addition, in normal cells the functions characteristic of the state of replication are shut off when the cells become quiescent again, and this may not happen in cancer cells, which may not enter a truly quiescent state. The considerable differences of gene expression between quiescent and growing cells suggest that stimulation of cell growth induces a new state of differentiation in the cells (growth-related differentiation).

WHAT CAUSES THE MAJORITY OF THE IRREGULARITIES OF GENE EXPRESSION IN CANCER CELLS?

Our thinking on this question is guided by recent results obtained in studies of viral and chemical carcinogenesis in experimental systems.

VIRAL CARCINOGENESIS

TRANSFORMING GENES. Work with several oncogenic viruses has shown that each causes cancer in animals or cell transformation in vitro through the expression of a single gene, the transforming gene.[12] With the Rous Sarcoma Virus of chicken temperature-sensitive mutations in this gene have a very dramatic effect: cells transformed by the mutant virus are transformed at a low temperature, when the gene is active but revert to normality after raising the temperature to inactivate the gene. The reversion occurs so rapidly that it must be due to an inactivation of the protein specified by the transforming gene. In fact, simply blocking protein synthesis causes the phenotype to change; and some of the changes occur in enucleated cells. These results show that transformation is caused by a rather unstable transforming protein, the product of the transforming gene.

This finding seems to create a paradox, because cells transformed by the Rous Sarcoma Virus are, like cancer cells, altered in many properties; therefore all the alterations must be attributed to the expression of a single gene. One possible explanation is that the transforming protein is pleiotropic and can affect many genes or their products.

The question about the nature and properties of the transforming protein has been solved by Erikson by isolating the transforming protein from transformed cells by immuno-

precipitation. He showed that this protein is the product
of the transforming gene by synthesizing an identical protein
in vitro using a cell-free system primed by the viral mRNA
that transcribes the gene. Then the combined efforts of
Erikson and Hunter showed that this protein has a peculiar
function; it is a protein kinase that phosphorylates tyrosine
in proteins (whereas other kinases phosphorylate serine or
threonine).[13,14]

THE MECHANISM OF TRANSFORMATION

How the Rous Sarcoma Virus transforms the cells is
still unclear. There arc two possibilities. One is that
transformation is caused by the protein kinase function, by
phosphorylating proteins important in the regulation of gene
expression. The other is that it is caused by the interaction of the transforming protein with the cell plasma
membrane, where it seems to be localized in the transformed
cells; the phosphorylating function would be needed for the
autoregulation of the protein. In fact it is well conceivable
that a protein interacting with the cell membrane may alter
the functions of many genes, as many polypeptide hormones and
growth factors do. In cells transformed by the Rous Sarcoma
Virus these alterations may be mainly due to the activation
of the growth-related differentiation state.
Studies with several other viruses, like polyoma virus,
or the Abelson Virus[15] have revealed that their transforming
proteins, although molecularly different, have a similar
protein kinase activity.

THE TRANSFORMING GENE IS A CELLULAR GENE

No matter what the precise mechanism of transformation
is, these results show that a single protein can alter many
cellular gene functions. Therefore, in principle, a cancer
may well be induced by a single deranged protein in a cell.
This generalization is legitimate because the transforming
gene of the Rous Sarcoma Virus is cellular, and is picked up
by the virus just as in generalized transduction with
bacteriophages. In fact, Bishop showed that radioactive
probes specific for the transforming gene present in the virus
hybridize to the DNA of uninfected chicken cells. The kinetics is compatible with the presence of one or few genes with
high homology to the viral genes in each cell; and a related
gene is present in other animal species. Both Erikson and
Bishop[16,17] found that the uninfected cells contain a
protein very similar in properties to that present in the
virus-infected cells. Moreover, Hanafusa showed that non-

transforming viral mutants -- in which the gene is partially deleted -- can pick up the missing part from cells by recombination, reacquiring both a complete gene and transforming ability.[18]

These results present us with another apparent paradox, because cells containing the transforming gene and the transforming protein may be perfectly normal. Lack of transformation in these cells can be explained in two ways. One explanation is the greater concentration (about ten times more) of the protein in the transformed cells, because the gene present in the virus is not regulated; another is that the gene is somewhat altered when it is picked up by the virus.

In either case we reach two important conclusions: 1) normal cells contain genes with the potential for inducing transformation; 2) transpositions of the gene to a virus allows it to transform the cells, presumably by increasing its expression by an order of magnitude. The implications of these results for cancer are clear: cancer can result from an event that activates a potential cancer gene always present in the cells by increasing its rate of expression. Conceivably this can be caused by genetic events of several kinds, such as mutations in a control region, or transposition of the gene to a chromatin segment that is normally expressed at a high rate.

CHEMICAL CARCINOGENESIS -- GENETIC EVENTS

A further understanding of the process by which cancer cells arise can be based on studies of chemical carcinogenesis. The first contribution of these studies is to clarify what the genetic event leading to cancer may be. Since more than half of all carcinogens can be shown to be mutagens,[19] or to generate mutagens after metabolic or chemical activation, mutations may be one of the genetic events of cancer. This concept is supported by the cancer-inducing effect of certain germinal mutations such as hereditary retinoblastoma, and by the abundance of skin cancers in xeroderma pigmentosum patients, in which ultraviolet light induces cancers owing to deficient DNA repair. Carcinogens also promote sister chromatids exchange; hence recombination or transposition of chromosomes may be another of the genetic events of cancer. Indeed in an increasing number of cancers characteristic chromosomal changes are being recognized cytologically using improved staining technologies.[20,21,22]

However about 30-40% of carcinogens are not mutagens or promutagens.[19] Therefore, other events must be involved in the activation of the potential cancer gene. What these events may be is shown by studies in several experimental systems.

REGULATION OF GENE EXPRESSION IN DEVELOPMENT

Before discussing the results relevant to the carcinogenic process, I must make a brief foray in the regulation
of gene expression of animal cells related to development.
An animal develops through a series of steps; in each step
a new set of genes becomes activated. This set may include
genes for specific products, genes controlling cell multiplication, and regulatory genes that respond to specific
environmental factors (such as hormones, growth factors, and
possibly contact with other cells). Certain genes may be
also active in cells at other or all steps of differentiation.
However, regulatory and growth control genes are probably
specific for each step.

INITIATION AND PROMOTION

The study of chemical carcinogenesis yields two
fundamental results relevant to the nature of oncogenetic
events important in cancer. One is that the outcome of the
administration of a certain dose of a carcinogen depends
very markedly on how it is administered.[23,24,25] Thus with
fast-acting carcinogens that do not linger around in the
body (e.g., N-nitrosomethylurea), a single application (or
two closely spaced applications) have little effect and only
result in some hyperplasia and a small proportion of benign
tumors. In contrast two or three well-spaced applications,
with a 3-4 week interval, produce a much higher incidence
of tumors, which are mostly malignant.[24] This shows that
certain cellular events following the first administration
strongly influence the outcome of subsequent administrations.
The other result is that in the mouse skin a single dose of
a carcinogen may be without noticeable effects, but a
subsequent long-term treatment with a promoting agent then
causes the appearance of tumors (usually papillomas).
Similar results are observed in other systems.
    The conclusion from these two observations is that
induction of tumors requires two events, as indicated more
than thirty years ago by Berenblum[26,27] and by Rous[28]: an
immediate irreversible event (initiation and subsequent
cellular events (promotion) that develop over a period of
weeks or months.

INITIATION

Initiation is almost certainly the genetic event discussed before. In fact many mutagens are initiators, and
the rate of initiation is increased if DNA replicates at the
time of the administration of the initiator, so that the DNA
damage can be fixed before it is repaired.[29]

PROMOTION

The nature of promotion is not as clear, but it can be
inferred from available evidence.

PROMOTION AND DIFFERENTIATION

Considerations on the nature of promotion is dominated
by considerations of the differentiation pattern[30] of the tissue
in which the tumor develops. Thus in the skin there is a
very regular series of steps in which a stem cell divides,
generating a clone of differentiated cells.[31,32] At the end of
the process the entire clone is discarded as squamous cells.
Initiation affecting any cell of the clone is irrelevant
because the cells are thrown out. And even initiation in a
stem cell may be irrelevant under normal conditions because
one of the products of division becomes again a quiescent
stem cell, whereas the other generates the throwaway clone.
Treatment with promoters (e.g., certain phorbol esters)
alters the situation profoundly by stimulating cell growth
and inhibiting differentiation.[33] Promoters cause skin hyperplasia. Under their influence presumably the stem cells
multiply without differentiating, and form stem cell clones;
a preexisting initiation in the original cell of such a clone
would cause the clone to grow into a tumor.
In this analysis there is a basic assumption: that
genetic cancer events are not expressed in quiescent cells, a
point to which I shall return.
In the mammary gland similar events happen although the
situation is somewhat different in detail. A chemical
initiator can produce a focal hyperplastic lesion (a hyperplastic alveolar module) if at the time of application, owing
to hormonal stimulation, the gland contains actively dividing
cells in ducts and alveoli.
Both ductal and alveolar cells replicate under appropriate hormonal stimulation. Whether among these dividing cells
there are separate stem cells is not clear.[34] The evolution of
cell types in the mammary gland is probably quite different
than in the skin, because the mammary gland, except for

lactation and weaning, is a conservative system in which
essentially all cells are retained. However, the principle
of carcinogenesis is the same: the formation, by differentiation, of clones of cells in which the changes of initiation
can be phenotypically expressed.

The initial tumors formed in both systems are benign,
essentially hyperplastic nodules (like the skin papillomas)
that have little of the derangement of cellular functions
present in cancer cells[27] Frequently these lesions are re-
versible if the promoting stimulus (chemical or hormonal) is
discontinued, showing that their existence depended on that
stimulus. Presumably the differentiation signals are
sufficiently strong when the promoting stimulus is removed to
restore normal cell renewal. However evidence also shows that
these lesions need the event of initiation.

Why should initiation be expressed only in a growing
clone, as I have assumed? I can suggest a hypothesis based
on the evolution of active genes in differentiation which I
already outlined. The model has two points: 1) genes that
after being damaged are able to cause the formation of an
initial neoplastic clone are those that affect growth regulation during the hyperplastic growth of cells; 2) these genes
are not expressed in quiescent cells or during the replace-
ment multiplication of stem cells.

MECHANISM OF THE DERANGEMENT OF GENE EXPRESSION IN CANCER --
ROLE OF PROMOTION

The next question is how the derangement of gene expression present in the cells of advanced cancers occurs.
The only guide we have on this question is that formation of
such cancers requires repeated applications of carcinogen (as
I already discussed) or the prolonged application of a tumor
promoter. In mammary carcinogenesis by N-nitrosomethylurea
in rat without promoting stimulus, a single injection of the
carcinogen induces generalized hyperplasia in the mammary
gland and, in time, benign tumors. The hyperplasia-inducing
activity of the carcinogen is probably the result of the
promoting activity of the carcinogen itself. Since, like
other carcinogens, NMU acts not only on DNA but also on RNA
and proteins[35] some of the altered non-DNA components may be
responsible for the promoting activity. This promotion may
occur by a mechanism of protein modification in a way related,
although not necessarily similar, to that observed with the
Rous Sarcoma Virus transforming protein. In time the effect
subsides, but in the meantime altered clones have the
opportunity to develop.

On the basis of these findings, repeated spaced injections of NMU can be considered equivalent to a summation of
repeated initiations in cells in which prolonged promotion
causes a continuing change of expressed genes. Progression
to increasing malignancy would be due to the effect of genetic
damages on a broader gene repertoire. Increased malignancy is
always the outcome, owing to selection for unregulated growth,
infiltration, metastasis; but many other independent changes,
not selected for, probably occur by the same mechanism and
generate the derangement of cellular functions characteristic
of cells of advanced cancers.

OTHER EVENTS IN PROGRESSIONS

In progression other phenomena may play a role in causing
the derangements of cellular functions. One such phenomenom
may be the preferential reaction of carcinogens with the DNA
of active chromatin.[36] In any given state of differentiation
of a cell, the genes of active chromatin are expressed or can
be induced to expression by suitable inducers. Stretches
containing these genes are recognizable by their high sensitivity to digestion with DNase I. Another phenomenon is
aneuploidization, since most advanced cancers and especially
their metastases are aneuploid. Aneuploidization may result
from alterations of proteins of the spindle following
modification or genetic rearrangement.

A MODEL FOR CARCINOGENESIS

In conclusion the complex nature of the cancer cells
reflects the complex nature of the process of carcinogenesis
and cannot be fully explained without a full understanding of
carcinogenesis itself. However in carcinogenesis only some
of the events are clear, others are understood in a general
way, whereas others must be hypothesized.
Chemical carcinogenesis of the mammary gland by NMU can
be interpreted by the following model, based on the previous
discussion.
1)   In the normal resting gland the cells express
"maintenance" genes. Initiators cannot induce neoplasias.
2)   A first injection of NMU causes initiations (genetic
events) and hyperplasia (a nongenetic event).
Hyperplasia is caused by the activation of some growth
control genes (promotion viewed essentially as the result of
protein modification); initiations that have occurred in these
genes are therefore revealed, causing focal, benign, histo-
logically typical neoplasias.

3) A second injection of NMU favors more extensive
initiations in control genes for growth-related differentiation because these genes were already expressed at the time
of injection and are therefore vulnerable. The carcinogen
also produces a second wave of promotion, which by modifying
proteins produced as a result of the first wave of promotion
changes further the expressed part of the genome. In unpre-
dictable ways some old genes may be shut off, others may be
activated. Initiations in newly activated genes may increase
malignancy.

4) A third injection of carcinogen renews and extends
the results of the second injection. Highly atypical cancers
may now be generated and progress.

This model can be applied to many cases of chemical
carcinogenesis. According to this model, carcinogenesis is
a Darwinian process in which initiation and promotion are the
driving evolutionary forces, the characteristics of the genome
providing the selective and restraining forces. Because
initiations occur at random the evolution of cancer cells
cannot be predicted in detail; however the general features
of cell evolution, deriving from the nature of the genes
involved, are predictable.

CONSEQUENCES OF THE MODEL

The model has interesting consequences, such as the
following:

1) In order to be also a carcinogen, a mutagen must be
able to induce promotion. For this reason mutagens that only
interact with DNA (such as 5-Bromodeoxyuridine) are not
carcinogenic by themselves. A promoting initiator can be
carcinogenic only if available to cells for a sufficiently
long time, because promotion must be prolonged.

2) The benign lesions induced by chemicals, or viruses,
which are often referred to as preneoplastic[37] may be truly so,
but only a fraction of them probably evolves to cancer. This
fraction may be small. Some may regress entirely.

3) Carcinogenesis in vivo can be duplicated only to a
limited extent in vitro, because the regulatory conditions
are so different in the two systems.

4) Induction of neoplasia by substances that cannot
initiate but are capable of altering the state of differentiation of the cells (such as ovarian hormones or zinc deficiency)[39] is due to their strong promoting action. Because
initiation without promotion may be entirely silent, it is
likely that promotion is the most important aspect of
carcinogenesis.

5) Differentiation is a strong inhibitor of a cancer phenotype: it prevents the formation of the cancer state and may cause its reversion.[40,41,42] Because of this inhibition, presumably only a tiny portion of initiations results in cancer.

6) The much smaller rate of cancer incidence per astronomical time in long-lived animals[43] (a requirement for long life) results mainly from differences in promotion. These have developed in evolution by complex changes in the organization of the animal genome. The changes may affect the proteins that, in the native state or after suitable modification, can cause promotion, the order of control genes in their spatial relation to targets for such proteins, the distribution of control and other genes, etc.

7) Carcinogenesis by viruses is also subject to promotion. The Rous Sarcoma Virus and a few other related viruses may be exceptional because they are very effective promoters causing a rapid shift to growth-related differentiation. In long-lived animals (like man) it may be unlikely to find oncogenic viruses of the same kind, i.e., that induce cancer alone. The expectation is that oncogenic human viruses will act as promoters able to act in concern with independent initiations.

8) The previous concepts suggest that assessment of the carcinogenic risk of chemical agents in humans is extremely difficult, for their promoting activity would have to be evaluated. Extrapolations to humans of effects obtained with high doses in rodents would not be justified because the same substance may not be an equally good promoter in both species and because the dose response for promotion need not be linear.

REFERENCES

1. Ibsen, K.H. and Fishman, W.H. *Biochimica et Biophysica Acta 560:* 243-280 (1979).
2. Lindahl, K.F. *Nature 280:* 105-106 (1979).
3. Bramwell, M.E. and Harris, H. *Proc R Soc Lond B 201:* 87-106 (1978).
4. Cikes, M. *Europ J Cancer 14:* 211-215 (1978).
5. Koyama, K., Nudelman, E., Fukuda, M., and Hakomon, S. *Cancer Research 39:* 3677-3682 (1979).
6. Murray, J.C., Liotta, L., Rennard, S.I., and Martin, G.R. *Cancer 40:* 347-351 (1980).
7. Buick, R.N., Stanisic, T.H., Fry, S.E., Salmon, S.E., Trent, J.M., and Krasovich, P. *Cancer Research 39:* 5051-5056 (1979).
8. Cifone, M.A. and Fidler, I.J. *Proc Natl Acad Sci USA 77:* 1039-1043 (1980).
9. Wang, B.S., McLoughlin, G.A., Richie, J.P., and Mannick, J.A. *Cancer Research 40:* 288-292 (1980).
10. Busch, H., Gyorkey, F., Busch, R.K., Davis, F.M., Gyorkey, P., and Smetana, K. *Cancer Research 39:* 3024-3030 (1979).
11. Wolfe, H.J. *New Eng J Med 299:* 146-147 (1978).
12. Vogt, P.K. *In:* H. Fraenkel-Conrat and R. Wagner (eds), *Comprehensive Virology.* Plenum Publishing Corp., New York (1977).
13. Collett, M.S. and Erikson, R.L. *Proc Natl Acad Sci USA 75:* 2021-2024 (1978).
14. Hunter, T. and Sefton, B.M. *Proc Natl Acad Sci USA 77:* 1311-1315 (1980).
15. Witte, O.N., Dasgupta, A., and Baltimore, D. *Nature 283:* 826-831 (1980).
16. Opperman, H., Levinson, A.D., Varmus, H.E., Levintow, L., and Bishop, J.M. *Proc Natl Acad Sci USA 76:* 1804-1808 (1979).
17. Collett, M.S., Brugge, J.S., and Erikson, R.L. *Cell 15:* 1363-1370 (1978).
18. Wang, L.H., Halper, C.C., Nadel, M., and Hanafusa, H. *Proc Natl Acad Sci USA 75:* 5812-5816 (1978).
19. Poirier, L.A. and de Serres, F.J. *J Natl Cancer Inst 62:* 919-926 (1979).
20. Kovacs, G. *Int J Cancer 21:* 688-694 (1978).
21. Sager, R. *Nature 282:* 447-448 (1979).
22. Wang, N., Trend, B., Bronson, D.L., and Fraley, E.E. *Cancer Research 40:* 796-802 (1980).
23. Topping, D.C., Griesemer, R.A., and Nettesheim, P. *Cancer Research 39:* 4823-4828 (1979).

24. Rose, D.P., Pruitt, B., Stauber, P., Ertürk, E., and Bryan, G.T. *Cancer Research 40:* 235-239 (1980).
25. Topping, D.C., Griesemer, R.A., and Nettesheim, P. *Cancer Research 39:* 4829-4837 (1979).
26. Berenblum, I. *Cancer Research 1:* 807-814 (1941).
27. Berenblum, I. and Shubik, P. *Brit J Cancer 3:* 384-386 (1949).
28. Friedenwald, W.F. and Rous, P. *J Exp Med 80:* 101-144 (1944).
29. Becker, F.F. *Cancer Research 39:* 5177-5178 (1979).
30. Cairns, J. *Nature 255:* 197-200 (1975).
31. Iversen, O.H., Bjerknes, R., and Devik, F. *Cell Tissue Kinet 1:* 351-367 (1968).
32. Potten, C.S. *Cell Tissue Kinet 7:* 77-88 (1974).
33. Weinstein, I.B., Wigler, M., and Pietropaolo, C. *In:* H.H. Hiatt, J.D. Watson, J.A. Kirston (eds.), *Origin of Human Cancer (Book B).* Cold Spring Harbor Laboratory, Cold Spring Harbor, New York, pp. 751-772 (1977).
34. Franke, W.W. and Keena, T.W. *Differentiation 13:* 81-88 (1979).
35. Miller, E.C. and Miller, J.A. *In:* A. Hollander (ed.), *Chemical Mutagens, Vol. 1.* Plenum Publishing Corp., New York, pp. 83-119 (1971).
36. Cox, R. *Cancer Research 39:* 2675-2678 (1979).
37. Medina, D., Oborn, C.J., and Asch, B.B. *Cancer Research 40:* 329-333 (1980).
38. Lemon, H.M. *Cancer 40:* 1825-1832 (1977).
39. Sivek, A. *Biochimica et Biophysica Acta 560:* 67-89 (1979).
40. Honma, Y., Kasukabe, T., Okabe, J., and Hozumi, M. *Cancer Research 39:* 3167-3171 (1979).
41. Pierce, G.B. and Wallace, C. *Cancer Research 31:* 127-134 (1971).
42. Pierce, G.B., Dixon, F.J., and Verney, E.L. *Lab Invest 9:* 583-602 (1960).
43. Peto, R. *In:* H.H. Hiatt, J.D. Watson, J.A. Kirsten (eds.) *Origin of Human Cancer (Book B).* Cold Spring Harbor Laboratory, Cold Spring Harbor, New York, p. 1403 (1977).

STUDIES ON POTENTIAL CARCINOGENS IN THE DIET OF INDIVIDUALS AT HIGH RISK FOR ESOPHAGEAL CANCER

MIN-HSIN LI

Institute of Cancer Research
Chinese Academy of Medical Science
Beijing, People's Republic of China

According to a nation-wide epidemiological survey on the mortality rates of cancer for the period 1973-1975 in China, Linxian County of Henan Province ranked first in the age-adjusted mortality rate of esophageal cancer, with 161.33/100,-000 in men and 102.88/1000,000 in women. There are several other high-risk areas, such as Yanzhong County in Jiangsu Province, Nan'os island on the border of Guangdong and Fukien Provinces, Langzhong County in the northern part of Sichuan Province, and Toli County in the Xinjian Uygur autonomous region.[1]

The populations in the different high-risk areas are separated from each other geographically, suggesting the importance of environmental factors in the development of esophageal cancer. In addition, in Linxian County the incidence rate and mortality rate of esophageal cancer increased gradually with age suggesting the accumulative effects of causal agents.[2] A positive relationship was noted between the contents of nitrates and nitrites in well water with the incidence of marked ephithelial dysplasia and carcinomas of the esophagus. Although the level of nitrates in the saliva of Linxian peasants is not higher than that found in peasants in Xingyang County of the same province, a low-risk area for esophageal cancer, the amount of urinary ascorbic acid in inhabitants of Linxian was only 1/8 to 1/9 that in Xinyang County peasants. In another study it was shown that the amount of nitrites excreted in the urine was markedly diminished following the administration of vitamin C. The low intake of vitamin C in Linxian might provide a favorable condition for the formation of nitrosamines from nitrites and secondary amines.[3,4]

Some foodstuffs in Linxian are frequently contaminated by Fusarium moniliforme and other fungi. We demonstrated the formation of dimethylnitrosamine (DMN), diethylnitrosamine (DEN), methylbenzylnitrosamine (MBN) and a new volatile N-nitroso compound, N-1-methylacetonyl-N-3-methylbutylnitrosamine (MAMBNA) in moldy cornbread after an 8-day incubation, when a small amount of $NaNO_2$ was added.

FIGURE 1

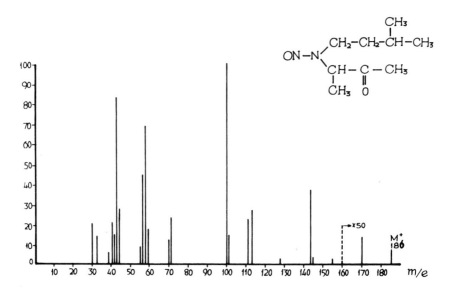

This new compound was obtained more often in Fusarium moniliforme inoculated cornbread. The 3-methylbutylamine radical of MAMBNS may be derived from leucine and isoleucine. It is known that maize flour is rich in leucine and isoleucine[5,6]. In eastern Africa and South Africa a high incidence of esophageal cancer was found in areas where maize was used as a staple food, and the consumption of alcoholic drinks made from maize was thought to be a possible etiological factor. Therefore our results may provide clues to the explanation of the high incidence of esophageal cancer in certain geographic areas where maize is consumed as the staple food.

We have done experimental studies in two groups of rats. In the first group, female rats were fed cornbread previously inoculated with Fusarium moniliforme. To each 400 gm sample of cornbread we also added 400 gm $NaNO_2$ and then incubated the material for 8 days. The presence of MAMBNA in cornbread was determined at regular intervals by thin-layer chromatography during the course of the experiment. Ten papillomas, 4 early carcinomas and one squamous cell carcinoma developed in the forestomach (an extention of the lower part of the esophagus) of 35 rats fed the moldy food. Most of the carcinomas were observed after 775 days of treatment. A second group of female rats were fed only the moldy

cornbread, i.e. without added $NaNO_2$. Two papillomas and 2
early carcinomas developed in the forestomach of 31 rats.
It should be noted that more papillomas and carcinomas were
induced in the first experimental group, indicating the combined effects of mycotoxins and nitrosamines. The control
group fed conventional cornbread had no tumors. These results provide evidence for the presence of nitrosamines and
mycotoxins in the moldy food. Our finding that chemical
carcinogens, in addition to mycotoxins, are formed in moldy
foodstuffs opens a new research field in cancer etiology.

TABLE 1

Carcinoma of the Forestomach in Rats Fed with
Fusarium Moniliforme Contaminated Cornbread*

Food	No. of rats in each group	No. of rats developing Lesions in the Forestomach**		
		Papilloma	Carcinoma	Mammary Tumors
F. moniliforme inoculated cornbread	31 ♀	2 (554, 596)	2 (621, 701)	4 (454–774)
F. moniliforme inoculated cornbread plus $NaNO_2$	35 ♀	10 (238–768)	5 (664–885)	4 (360–838)
Uninoculated cornbread	10 ♀	—	— (330–700)	—

*   Epithelial hyperplasia was observed in the lower portion of the esophagus and in the
glandular stomach of some experimental rats.

** Numbers in parenthesis are days after initiation of feeding when lesion was detected.

We also noted the development of mammary tumors in 8 experimental rats, probably due to the influence of mycotoxins
produced by Fusarium fungi that have estrogenic activity, such
as zearalenone.

Further studies on enhancement of formation of nitrosamines by fungi have been carried out: (1) as in certain
species of bacteria, some fungi, such as Fusarium moniliforme
can reduce nitrates to nitrites; (2) fungi contained in the

pickled vegetable from Linxian can also reduce nitrates to
nitrites, high levels are reached after 4 to 5 days of incubation, and this reducing action is lost after steam disin-
fection; (3) when cornbread was inoculated with a common
species of fungus encountered in Linxian, a marked increase
in content of secondary amines was noted, especially after
a 4-day incubation, a 17-fold increase in secondary amines
occurred in cornbread contaminated with Fusarium moniliforme;
and (4) Geotrichum candidum, the predominant fungus found
in pickled vegetables, can reduce nitrates to nitrites, increase the amount of secondary amines and enhance the formation of nitrosamines[8].

Concerning the pickled vegetables commonly consumed in
Linxian, in our previous work we observed the development of
an adenocarcinoma of the glandular stomach and other tumors
in rats following prolonged feeding of an extract of the concentrated juice. These results provide evidence for the
presence of carcinogens in pickled vegetables form Linxian
County, but its chemical nature remains to be identified[9].

From a dichloromethane extract of pickles vegetables we
isolated, identified and synthesized the nitroso compound
Roussin red methylester (Dimethanethiolatotetranitrosodiiron),
which was first synthesized by J. Roussin in 1858, although
it has not been reported to exist in natural products.[10]

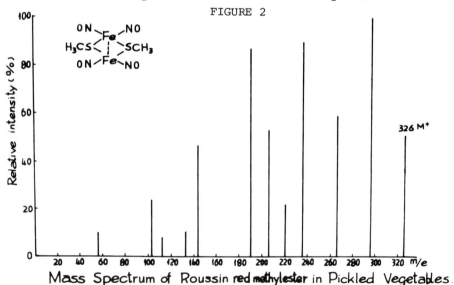

FIGURE 2

Mass Spectrum of Roussin red methylester in Pickled Vegetables.

This compound induced some papillomas of the forestomach in
mice after administration by gastric intubation for more
than 200 days. The experiment is still in progress, however,

and the tumorigenic effect of this compound is not stronger than the concentrated pickled vegetables.

A series of short-term tests have shown that extracts of pickled vegetables exerted mutagenic, cell-transforming and promoting activities in cell culture.

Furthermore, our recent studies show that a cyclohexane extract of pickled vegetables contains benzo(a)pyrene (BaP) and some other polycyclic aromatic hydrocarbon (PAH) compounds. Thin-layer chromatography analysis revealed the presence of BaP and PAH fluorescence bands. This was confirmed by spectrofluorometric determination (emission and excitation spectra).

In summary, our studies on etiological agents of esophageal cancer in the high-risk area indicate that environmental factors play an important role in the development of this malignant disease. In fungus-contaminated food we found potential carcinogens such as nitrosamines, mycotoxins, BaP and PAH. The carcinogencity of Roussin red in pickled vegetables remains to be studied. There are also several contributing factors in the environment. These include: nutritional deficiencies for animal proteins and fat; vitamins A, B_2 and C; high level of nitrates and nitrites in water and food; low molybdenum, zinc and imbalance of trace elements; as well as indoor air pollution from coal stoves during the winter months. The combined action of potential dietary carcinogens and these contributing factors may account for the prevalence of esophageal cancer in high-risk areas of the People's Republic of China.

REFERENCES

1. *Atlas of Cancer Maps of the People's Republic of China.*
    To be published in 1980.
2. The Coordinating Group for Res. Etiology of Esophageal
    Cancer of N. China. *Scientia Sinica, 18:*131-148, 1975.
3. Dept. Chem. Etiology and Carcinogenesis, Cancer Inst.,
    Chinese Acad. Med. Sci. *Adv. Med. Oncology Res. and
    Education, 3:*39-44, 1979.
4. Li, M.H., Li, P.J. *Adv. Cancer Res.,* 1980 (to be
    published).
5. Li, M.H., Lu, S.H., Ji, C., Wang, M., Cheng, S., Jiu, C.
    *Scientia Sinica, 22:*471-477, 1979.
6. Lu, S.H., Li, M.H., Ji, C., Wang, M., Wang, Y., Huang, L.
    *Ibid. 22:*601-608, 1979.
7. Li, M.H., Lu, S.H., Ji.C., Wang, M., Cheng, S., Tian, G.
    Z., *10th Int. Sym. Princess Takamatsu Cancer Res. Fund,*
    Abstract pp. 27-29, Japan, 1979.
8. Lu, S.H., Wang, Y., Li, M.H. *Acta Acad. Med. Sinicae, 2*
    (in Chinese). In press, 1980.
9. Dept. Chem. Etiology and Carcinogenesis, Cancer Inst.,
    Chinese Acad. Med. Sci. *Res. Cancer Treatment and Con-
    trol.* 1977 *(2):*46-49, 1977 (in Chinese).
10. Wang, G.H., Chang, W.X., Chai, W.G. *Chinese J. Chem.,*
    1980 (to be published).

ASSOCIATION OF THE EPSTEIN-BARR VIRUS
WITH NASOPHARYNGEAL CARCINOMA

WERNER HENLE, M.D.
GERTRUDE HENLE, M.D.
The Joseph Stokes, Jr.,
Research Institute of The Children's
Hospital of Philadelphia,
and the
School of Medicine
University of Pennsylvania
Philadelphia, Pennsylvania 19104

The first observation suggesting an association of the Epstein-Barr virus (EBV) with nasopharyngeal carcinoma (NPC) was made by chance. The virus was first detected by Epstein and his associates on electron microscopic examination within a small proportion of cells cultured from African Burkitt's lymphomas. When Lloyd Old and his associates at the Sloan-Kettering Institute showed that many sera from Burkitt's lymphoma (BL) patients gave one or more lines of precipitation in double diffusion precipitation tests with extracts of cultured BL cells, they requested and received control sera from African patients with other tumors. Among them were sera from NPC patients, and only these, but none of the other control sera, reacted, as had the BL sera, in the precipitation test.[1]

At that time, my wife and I had developed an immunofluorescence test for the detection of EBV in the BL cultures and for the titration of antibodies to the virus.[2] We found that NPC sera sent by Dr. Old and others had, like the BL sera, substantially higher titers of antibodies to EBV than any of the control sera.[3] Consequently, the geometric mean antibody titer of NPC patients was about 10-fold higher as compared to that seen in patients with other tumors.

Subsequently, the causal relation of EBV to infectious mononucleosis (IM) was found - again by a bit of chance - when one of our technicians developed this disease.[4] She had no previous antibodies to EBV but seroconverted in the course

Work by the authors has been supplied by research grant CA-04568 and contract NO1-CP-3-3272 from the National Cancer Institute, U. S. Public Health Service.

of her illness. This initial clue has been amply confirmed, and EBV is now generally accepted as the cause of IM.

Antibodies measured in the original immunofluorescence test turned out to be directed against viral capsid antigen (VCA), which is present in every virus-producing cell. We then found that virus from a producer culture of BL cells, when used to expose non-producer cultures, induced in the infected cells only an abortive cycle of viral replication with synthesis of two early antigens, the diffuse (D) and the restricted (R) components, but not of VCA and thus no virus particles.[5] Antibodies to the early antigens turned out to be largely disease-related, as we will discuss below. Like antibodies to VCA, they are titrated by the indirect immunofluorescence technique, which also permits to differentiate between the immunoglobulin class of the antibodies. The fourth antigen is the EBV-associated nuclear antigen (EBNA), discovered by Reedman and Klein[6], which is present in every EBV-transformed cell. Its detection in a cell thus proves that the cell carries EBV genomes. It is only possible to detect this by the very sensitive anti-complement immunofluorescence method. In addition, there are several EBV-determined cell membrane antigens, which are detectable on live cells; however, the techniques for measuring the corresponding antibodies are too complex for general use.

With these techniques, each of the EBV-associated diseases reveals a characteristic antibody pattern.[7] In acute infectious mononucleosis, one finds high IgM and IgG antibody titers to VCA, a transient antibody response to D, no antibodies as yet to EBNA, and usually heterophil antibodies of the Paul-Bunnell type. Primary EBV infections in infants under 2 years of age usually remain silent: as a rule there is no heterophil antibody response, and antibodies to the early antigen complex are directed against R rather than against D.[8] In the course of primary EBV infection, a viral carrier state becomes regularly established in the lymphoreticular system. This persistent latent infection is responsible for the lifelong maintenance, at moderate levels, of IgG antibodies to VCA and EBNA. It is rare when antibodies to early antigens persist, and then do so only when relatively high antibody titers to VCA are maintained. In Burkitt's lymphoma, high titers of antibodies to R are the outstanding feature, whereas in nasopharyngeal carcinoma, high D-specific IgG titers and, especially, high IgA antibody titers to VCA and D are characteristic.[9] The test for IgA antibodies to VCA and D turned out to be highly useful in the diagnosis and prognosis of NPC, as we shall discuss shortly.

These patterns do not often hold for their initial
stages of the diseases, but rather for the relatively
advanced cases of the tumor, because the antibody titers
depend to a considerable extent on the total tumor burden.
Also, after successful therapy the pattern may gradually
change toward the pattern seen in healthy individuals a long
time after primary EBV infections.[10] Finally, the usually
controlled viral carrier state established regularly in the
course of primary infections, may become upset by immuno-
suppressive diseases or therapy, then, antibody patterns are
evoked which can resemble those seen in BL or NPC. Thus, IgA
antibodies are found occasionally, but usually at low titers
in patients with Burkitt's lymphoma or other tumors and in
healthy individuals who maintain relatively high IgG antibodies.

For these reasons, it has long been necessary to provide
additional evidence for an association of EBV with either BL
or NPC. Such evidence has been forthcoming. The general
approaches used for linking a virus with a human malignancy
have been (a) detection of viral fingerprints (antigens,
nucleic acid) in the tumor; (b) malignant transformation of
normal cells by the virus in vitro; (c) induction of tumors
in non-human primates or other animals by injection of the
virus; and (d) demonstration of a broader spectrum and higher
titers of antibodies to virus-related antigens in patients
as compared to controls and their relation to the prognosis
of the patients.

As far as the second and third approaches are concerned,
limited efforts with probably inappropriate techniques have
been negative thus far; no epithelial cells have been found
infectible and transformable in vitro, and no carcinomas have
been induced in non-human primates. In contrast, EBV transforms primate lymphocytes in vitro into permanently growing
EBNA positive lymphoblasts and induces lymphomas in marmosets.
This supports a causal relationship of EBV to Burkitt's
lymphoma. The transformed cells and the lymphomas so obtained
do not entirely conform however to Burkitt's lymphomas.

The first approach, the detection of EB viral fingerprints has been successful. Viral DNA and EBNA-positive
carcinoma cells are found at high degrees of frequency in NPC
biopsies.[11,12,13] In one study on African patients with NPC
or other carcinomas biopsies were tested for EBV DNA in
George Klein's laboratory in Stockholm[14] and in another study
on Chinese patients with NPC or other carcinomas seen in Hong
Kong, touch preparations were made from biopsies and then sent
to Philadelphia for EBNA staining.[13] Undifferentiated or
poorly differentiated NPCs regularly contained EBV DNA in

amounts equivalent to multiple viral genomes per cell. If
the tumors showed some degree of differentiation, they were
no longer usually positive. None of the other carcinomas or
other tumors were positive. Similarly, almost all NPC
biopsies contained EBNA-positive carcinoma cells; in a few
specimens, however, either no tumor cells had been deposited
on the slides, or EBNA had escaped from the nucleus due to
necrosis. None of the other carcinomas showed EBNA positive
cells, except for undifferentiated carcinomas of the nasal
fossa, which arise adjacent to the usual site of NPC and
therefore may have the same origin. This technique is helpful in cases of lymph node metastases but unknown primary
site of the carcinoma. EBNA positive carcinoma cells in the
invaded lymph node clearly identify the postnasal space as
the primary site of the tumor. Similar results have been
obtained now in other parts of the world.[16,17,18]

To return to the EBV-specific serology, the IgG antibody
titers to VCA and the incidence and titers of IgG antibodies
to D clearly increase with the stage of the disease - i.e.,
the total tumor burden.[10] Similarly, the incidence and titers
of IgA antibodies to VCA and D increase from stage I to stage
IV (or formerly V).[9]

What goes up with the tumor burden should come down,
after the tumor has been successfully eradicated. This
turned out to be the case as shown in a 5-year follow-up
study of patients in Hong Kong.[19] There were over 100 NPC
patients who could be divided into 3 main groups. The first
which comprised more than half of the patients, showed no
relapses of the tumor, as well as gradual decline of all
antibodies to lower (anti-VCA IgG) or even nondetectable
levels (all other antibodies). In contrast, patients who
only responded temporarily to therapy (the second group of
about 30% of the patients) showed an upward trend of the
titers of some or all of the antibodies tested. Most remark-
ably, the antibody titers often rose months in advance of
clinical detection of recurrent tumors at the primary site
or in lymph nodes, or of the detection of widespread
metastases. The third group (about 15% of the patients)
showed an initial decline in all or some antibody titers, and
a subsequent reversal of this trend to a renewed broadening
of the antibody spectrum and increased antibody titers. Again,
the rises in antibody titers were noted well in advance of
clinical detection of renewed tumor activity.

These observations denote that the EBV-specific serology
may serve to monitor the effectiveness of therapy and to
forewarn of imminent relapses or metastases well before they
have become clinically evident. Therefore, rising antibody

titers should lead to an intensified search for the site of renewed tumor activity, and, if this is found, to an early reinstitution of therapy.

There are some exceptions to the general patterns, as here, in the remaining 5% of the patients. When the tumor invades the central nervous system by direct extension from the primary site without significant involvement of lymph nodes, there may be no substantial increases in antibody titers because the tumor burden remains small, except for the very final stage.

It is clear that NPC is not an immediate consequence of primary EBV infections. There is, in fact, an interval of many years - and even several decades - between the primary infection and the emergence of NPC. Under crowded living conditions, as in Hong Kong and other Chinese cities, primary EBV infections generally occur under the age of 5, yet the peak incidence of NPC occurs in the fifth decade of life.

Since NPC is apparently a monoclonal tumor,[20] the EBV genomes must have been present in the very first malignantly transformed nasopharyngeal epithelial cell. Infection of the tumor after its inception is precluded by the presence of circulating antibodies to the virus. Indeed, sera were found by Dr. Lanier in collections obtained for various purposes from Alaskan natives; the discovery of the sera was made between 2 and 10 years before the diagnosis of NPC. In as yet unpublished assays, 6 of these sera yielded antibody patterns within the range of those seen in healthy individuals well past primary EBV infection. There were no hints to alert us to the eventual fate of the serum donors.

In contrast, the seventh serum, gave an antibody pattern clearly indicative of NPC 17 months before diagnosis of the tumor. This patient sought medical aid when he was already in stage IV of NPC and died within 6 months. Since he had noticed lumps in his neck many months before, it is likely that he already had NPC when the early blood was drawn. Thus, if the EBV-specific serologic tests had been carried out then, there would have been an earlier diagnosis of his disease leading to earlier, and perhaps more successful, therapy.

By now the test for IgA antibodies to VCA has been used, with some modification, in mass surveys conducted during 1978 and 1979 in the People's Republic of China. We have had remarkable results in the early detection of NPC, which Dr. Li Chen Ch'uan will present in detail during this conference.

There remain many unsolved problems. Foremost among them, we do not know as yet how, the EBV genomes become associated with the carcinoma cells. It is possible that

renewed efforts will reveal epithelial cells in the nasopharynx, which are infectible and transformable by EBV.
Another possible way to introduce EBV genomes into nasopharyngeal epithelial cells would be by their fusion with
enveloped EB virus particles or of EBV genome-carrying
lymphocytes during respiratory infections by parainfluenza
or other viruses known to cause fusion of cells. Such fusion
of cultured Burkitt's lymphoma cells has been achieved in
vitro with HeLa cells, but not as yet with normal epithelial
cells. This hypothesis also might be testable in non-human
primates by simultaneous intranasal inoculation of both EBV
and a parainfluenza virus.

It is most likely that, in addition to EBV, a number of
other factors play important roles in the development of NPC.
Among the Chinese, there is clear genetic disposition, as
evidenced by multiple cases spanning several generations in
given families; also, with the decrease, there is a frequent
association of a particular HLA type (Singapore-2) in Malaya,
which has not been found to be the case elsewhere in the
world. Inhalation or ingestion of carcinogens, such as nitrosamines, and nutritional deficiencies of vitamin A, are
considered among other contributing factors. Finally,
hormonal and immunological factors could well influence the
emergence of the tumor.

REFERENCES

1. Old, J.L., Boyse, E.A., Oettgen, H.F., deHarven, E.,
    Geering, G., Williamson, B., and Clifford, P.: Precipita-
    ting antibody in human serum to an antigen present in
    cultured Burkitt's lymphoma cells. *Proc. Nat. Acad. Sci.
    (USA) 56:* 1699-1704, 1966.
2. Henle, G., and Henle, W.: Immunofluorescence in cells
    derived from Burkitt's lymphoma. *J. Bact. 91:* 1248-1256,
    1966.
3. Henle, W., Henle, G., Ho H.C., Burtin, P., Cachin, Y.,
    Clifford, P., deSchryver, A., de-The, G., Diehl, V., and
    Klein, G.: Antibodies to EB virus in nasopharyngeal
    carcinoma, other head and neck neoplasms and control
    groups. *J. Nat. Cancer Inst. 44:* 225-231, 1970.
4. Henle, G., Henle, W., and Diehl, V.: Relation of Burkitt
    tumor associated herpes-type virus to infectious mono-
    nucleosis. *Proc. Nat. Acad. Sci. (USA) 59:* 94-101, 1968.
5. Henle, G., Henle, W., and Klein, G.: Demonstration of
    two distinct components in the early antigen complex of
    Epstein-Barr virus infected cells. *Int. J. Cancer 8:*
    272-282, 1971.

6. Reedman, B.M., and Klein, G.: Cellular localization of an EBV-associated complement-fixing antigen in producer and non-producer lymphoblastoid cell lines. *Int. J. Cancer 11:* 499-520, 1973.

7. Henle, W., Henle, G., and Horwitz, C.A.: Epstein-Barr virus-specific diagnostic tests in infectious mononucleosis. *Human Pathologh 5:* 551-565, 1974.

8. Biggar, R.J., Henle, G., Boocker, J., Lennette, E.T., Fleisher, G., and Henle, W.: Primary Epstein-Barr virus infections in African infants. II. Clinical and serological observations during seroconversion. *Int. J. Cancer 22:* 244-250, 1978.

9. Henle, G., and Henle, W.: Epstein-Barr virus-specific IgA serum antibodies as an outstanding feature of nasopharyngeal carcinoma. *Int. J. Cancer 17:* 1-7, 1976.

10. Henle, W., Ho, H.C., Henle, G., and Kwan, H.C.: Antibodies to Epstein-Barr virus-related antigens in nasopharyngeal carcinoma. Comparison of active cases and long term survivors. *J. Nat. Cancer Inst. 51:* 361-369, 1973.

11. zurHausen, H., Schulte-Holthausen, H., Klein, G., Henle, W., Henle, G., Clifford, P., and Santesson, L.: EB-virus DNA in biopsies of Burkitt tumors and anaplastic carcinomas of the nasopharynx. *Nature 228:* 1056-1058, 1970.

12. Wolf, H., zurHausen, H., Klein, G., Becker, V., Henle, G., and Henle, W.: Attempts to detect virus-specific DNA sequences in human tumors. III. Epstein-Barr viral DNA in non-lymphoid nasopharyngeal carcinoma cells. *Med. Microbiol. Immunol. 161:* 15-21, 1975.

13. Huang, D.P., Ho, J.H.C., Henle, W., and Henle, G.: Demonstration of EBV-associated nuclear antigens in NPC cells from fresh biopsies. *Int. J. Cancer 14:* 580-588, 1974.

14. Andersson-Anvret, M., Forsby, N., Klein, G., and Henle, W.: Studies on the occurrence of Epstein-Barr virus-DNA in nasopharyngeal carcinomas, in comparison with tumors of other head and neck regions. *Int. J. Cancer 20:* 486-494, 1977.

15. Huang, D.P., Ho, H.C., Henle, W., Henle, G., Saw, D., and Lui, M.: Presence of EBNA in nasopharyngeal carcinoma and control patient tissues related to EBV serology. *Int. J. Cancer 22:* 266-274, 1978.

16. DeSchryver, A., Klein, G., Henle, W., and Henle, G.: EB virus-associated antibodies in Caucasian patients with carcinoma of the nasopharynx and in long-term survivors after treatment. *Int. J. Cancer 13:* 319-325, 1974.

17. Andersson-Anvret, M., Forsby, N., Klein, G., Henle, W., and Bjorklund, A.: Relationship between the Epstein-Barr virus genome and nasopharyngeal carcinoma in Caucasian patients. *Int. J. Cancer 23*: 762-767, 1979.

18. Lanier, A., Talbot, M., Clift, S., Tschopp, C., Dohan,P., Bornkamm, G., and Henle, W.: Epstein-Barr virus DNA in tumor tissue from native Alaskan patients with naso-pharyngeal carcinoma. *Lancet 2*: 1095, 1978.

19. Henle, W., Ho, H.C., Henle, G., Chau, J.C.W., and Kwan, H.C.: Nasopharyngeal carcinoma: Significance of changes in Epstein-Barr virus-related antibody patterns follow-ing therapy. *Int. J. Cancer 20*: 663-672, 1977.

20. Fialkow, P.J., Martin, G.M., Klein, G., Clifford, P., and Singh, S.: Evidence for a clonal origin of head and neck tumors. *Int. J. Cancer 9*: 133-142, 1972.

ASPECTS OF RESEARCH STUDIES
ON LIVER CARCINOMA

YAO ZHEN
Shanghai Institute of Cell Biology
Academia Sinica

As you know, the incidence of hepatocellular carcinoma
is relatively high in China, amounting to 50 per hundred
thousand in some high-risk areas. Due to this high incidence,
together with difficulty in its early diagnosis and poor
prognosis, hepatoma becomes one of our most serious types of
cancer. Basic research studies on liver carcinoma in China
during the past twenty years has been recently reviewed.[1]
I would like to take this opportunity to summarize some of
our own works, which include studies with human liver
carcinoma and rat hepatoma.

IN VITRO CULTURED HUMAN LIVER CARCINOMA CELL LINES

In 1960 Professor Chen and his colleagues succeeded in
establishing in vitro the first human hepatoma cell line.
In 1974, they further established three such cell lines,
designated as BEL-7402, 7404 and 7405.

The biological characteristics of these cell lines were
summarized in a recent paper by these authors.[2] In short,
they are hypotriploid cell lines with a model chromosome
number about 60 and an abnormally large acrocentric chromosome.
The epithelial nature of these cell lines was proved by the
presence of desmosomes and tonofibrils. AFP was detected
intracellularly, and LDH G6PD and TAT enzyme activities were
found to be similar to those of primary liver tumors.

The marker chromosome was not directly searched for in
clinical specimens, but was found to be absent in the primary
outgrowths of epithelial-like cells from cultured fragments
of another three surgical samples between 1-16 transfers.
However, some points of interest were obtained by G-banding
study of chromosomes of human hepatoma from the latter
material[3]: 1) acrocentric chromosomes of D and G groups
tended to decrease in number and monosomy as well as nullisomy
of the chromosome 15 were found in 90% of tumor cells
analyzed. Chromosomes 21 and 22 were also reduced in number
in 23-33% of cells analyzed; 2) metacentric or submetacentric
E and F group chromosomes tended to increase in number,

generally reaching hypotetraploid, or even forming octosomy
in many tumor cells. More case analyses are needed to determine whether chromosome imbalance created by the excess of E
and F group chromosomes over those of G and D groups, or the
existence of monosomy or nullisomy of particular chromosomes
is a consequence of short-term in vitro cultivation or is, in
some way, associated with malignant transformation of liver
cells.

The established human hepatoma cell lines - BEL-7402,
-7404 and -7405 - are now being used as experimental system
for the studies of human liver carcinoma, with particular
emphasis on gene expression and its regulation by methods of
somatic cell genetics and other related techniques.

FETAL ANTIGENS IN HUMAN LIVER CARCINOMA

It is well known that embryonic gene products are expressed by most animal and human cancer cells and that they
may be utilized as biological markers of malignant diseases.
Such antigens as well as ectopic hormones, enzymes and other
biochemical products, have been the subject of many recent
international conferences.[4-5] In 1970, we began to adopt
the use of α-fetoprotein, originally developed by Abelev and
Tatarinov,[6] for clinical diagnosis of hepatoma. We isolated
this protein from sera of hepatoma patients and developed the
sensitive radioimmunoassay method; in 1971, for the first
time in China, we also succeeded in using immunodiffusion
test of AFP for mass screening. In a total of 921 workers
examined in one district area in Shanghai, we found two cases
of early hepatoma without any positive indication by the
methods of diagnosis which were then available, such as
ultrasonic and radioisotope scannings and blood enzyme tests.
Surgical exploration of one of the two patients revealed a
small nodule of hepatocellular carcinoma of the size of
2.5x3 cm. Since then, more sensitive reverse haemagglutina-
tion assay and radio-rocket electrophoresis were developed
by other institutions and used in mass surveys in high-risk
areas, and the value of AFP screening in the detection of
early hepatoma was fully confirmed.[7]

However, since about 10% of hepatoma patients are AFP
negative and since, among the so-called low AFP titer individuals (blood AFP level 40-200ng/ml) arising from mass
screening, there is no reliable means of detection which could
be used to differentiate those very early hepatomas from the
rest of liver diseases therefore, we have looked for other
possible markers. We have found that cultured human hepatoma
cells possessed a membrane-associated fetal antigen, cross-

reactive to fetal liver cells. This was demonstrated by both the immunofluorescence and immunoferritin methods as described in our previous papers.[8,9]

In both these experiments, anti-AFP and anti-CEA sera were used as controls, and immunoelectrophoresis and cross-immunoelectrophoresis were also run with immunofluorescent positive serum toward related antigens. The results indicated that this membrane-associated antigen is neither AFP nor CEA.

In fetal liver there are two kinds of cells, namely, hepatocytes and haemopoietic cells at various stages of differentiation. Both of these types of cells gave positive reaction. Moreover, fetal lung, kidney and heart cells also reacted to the positive antiserum to a lesser degree. Thus, this fetal antigen did not appear to be an organ-specific liver fetal antigen.

In order to make sure that the fetal antigen observed was not an artifact introduced by fetal calf serum or an induced expression by some contaminated virus, we have used the unlabeled immunoperoxidase technique* to localize such antigen in surgical specimens of primary hepatomas. Table 1 listed the results of this immunocytochemical study. In twenty-two fetal livers at different developmental stages, hepatocytes of 3-4 month fetuses gave much stronger membrane and cytoplasmic reaction than those of 5-7 month fetuses. This might suggest the phasic nature of the antigen, which was, however, not investigated in detail. All surgical specimens of hepatomas showed definite positive reaction with varying intensities on cell surface and in the cytoplasm, while five biopsy specimens of normal liver exhibited negative reaction under identical conditions.[10] These preliminary results suggest that the antigen is another oncofetal antigen common to various individual hepatomas (Table 1, Figs. 1-4).

The lack of organ specificity of this fetal antigen was also indicated through limited examination of the reaction of other human tumors. Some lung, colon and rectal carcinomas studied thus far have all shown positive cytoplasmic reaction without significant membrane staining. Nevertheless, the reaction of several cirrhotic livers appeared to be negative; however more analysis is needed before we can be sure that this antigen is absent from regenerating and inflammatory liver tissues.

Our attempts to isolate this fetal antigen met with limited success. Solubilization of this antigen was made by

* We would like to express our gratitude to Professor Konrad C. Hsu of Columbia University for establishing this PAP method when he visited and lectured in our institute in 1978.

TABLE 1

Cases of specimens	Histo-pathological classification	Blood fetoprotein	Immunoperoxidase reaction		
	Distribution of fetal antigen in human primary hepatoma cells			membrane	cytoplasm	nucleus
1	Mixed hepato-biliary carcinoma	+	+	±	-
2	Hepato cellular carcinoma, grade II	+	+	+	-
3	Hepatocellular carcinoma, grade II	-	+	+→++	-
4	Hepatocellular carcinoma, grade II	+	+	±	-
5	Mixed hepato-biliary carcinoma	+	+	±	-
6	Hepatocellular carcinoma, grade III	+	++	+	-
7	Hepatocellular carcinoma	+	+	+	-
8	Hepatocellular carcinoma, grade II	+	++	±	-
9	Hepatocellular carcinoma, grade II	+	++	+	-
10	Hepatocellular carcinoma, grade III	+	±	±	-
Fetal liver cells, age about 3 months		+	++	+	-

-, Negative; ±, Weakly positive; +, Positive; ++, Strongly positive
(Reprinted, with permission, from Shi et al, paper submitted to publication)

FIGURE 1

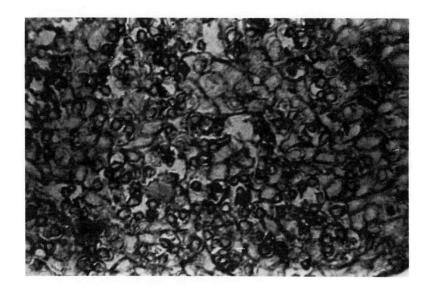

FIGURE 2

FIGURE 3

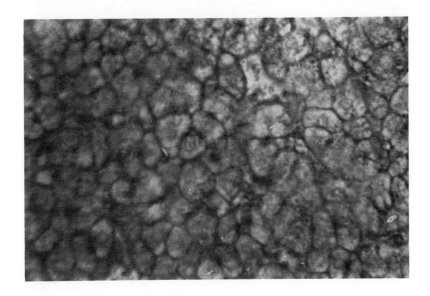

FIGURE 4

3M KCL extraction from fetal liver cells and BEL-7402 hepatoma cells. Rabbit antisera to these extracts were purified by immunoabsorption chromatography on sepharose 4B, coupled with a mixture of equal amounts of 3M KCL extract of adult liver cells and normal serum proteins and finally absorbed with mixed white blood cells. This absorbed serum was used to monitor the different fractions of extracted antigen column-chromatographed on ultragel ACA 54, using the quenching of indirect membrane immunofluorescence as an indicator. Active fractions were found in the first and third elution peaks.[11] Further purification of this antigen by Con-A-sepharose and WGA-sepharose is still under investigation.

LOCALIZATION OF SURFACE AND CORE ANTIGEN OF HEPATITIS B VIRUS IN HUMAN HEPATOMA

In recent years, the presence of antibodies to hepatitis B virus surface and core antigen in the sera of hepatoma patients has been reported by many authors. The production of HBsAg by a human hepatoma cell line has also been demonstrated. All of this evidence suggests the possible role of hepatitis-B virus in the etiology of human hepatoma. However, there are very few reports of the in situ localization of these antigens in hepatoma cells. Recently, some of our colleagues examined the cellular localization of HBsAg and HBcAg in primary hepatocellular carcinomas by immunoperoxidase technique.[12] The results demonstrated the presence of both antigens in the cells in what appear to be noncancerous areas of tissue, but only HBsAg was found in hepatoma cells. The intracellular localization of these two antigens was the same as in liver cells, cases of hepatitis, i.e., HBsAg only localized in the cytoplasm and only HBcAg in the nucleus.

CELL-MEDIATED CYTOTOXICITY AND IMMUNE RNA STUDIES IN HUMAN HEPATOMA

We have some indirect evidence suggesting the possible presence of tumor-associated antigen in human hepatomas and of immune response in hepatoma patients. When BEL-7402 cells were labeled with ^{125}IUdR, in vitro cell cytotoxicity tests indicated that out of 33 hepatoma patients, peripheral blood lymphocytes in 13 of them (40%) showed definite cytotoxic activity. Most of these cases (11/13) were stage II hepatomas, and half of them (6/13) had a decrease in AFP level after surgical removal of the tumors. Among 20 cases whose peripheral blood lymphocytes did not show any significant cytotoxic reaction, 15 of them were stage III, that is, advanced clinical cases with ascites and jaundice. This is what one

would expect from the general immune status of these patients.
However, the specificity of this microcytotoxicity reaction
was not tested with other tumor cell lines, nor was an attempt
made to study cell-mediated cytotoxicity of these patients'
lymphocytes to short-term cultures of their autologuous
hepatoma target cells.

On the other hand, we have demonstrated the mediation
of immune cytolysis of BEL-7402 cells in vitro by xenogenic
immune RNA, isolated from spleen and lymph nodes of sheep
immunized with BEL-7402 cells previously incubated with sheep
anti-human liver cell antiserum. When assayed with wheat germ
cell-free system, such I-RNAs were active for the increase of
uptake of labeled amino acids into the system. Nonimmune
human peripheral blood lymphocytes were converted into cytotoxic cells after incubation with such I-RNA. Enzyme treatment controls indicated the specificity of action of RNA in
this in vitro mediation.[14]

On this basis, we have also made some preliminary trials
with xenogenic I-RNA as a form of immunotherapy in combination
with other therapeutic measures for hepatoma patients. These
patients had had their primary tumors surgically removed, but
the chance of recurrence of the disease within 1 or 2 years
was very high. Our intention was to delay the relapse. At
the first application, 10 mg of I-RNA was incubated at $37^{o}C$
with exudate cells (mainly macrophages and granulocytes) isolated from a dermal blister following the application of
cantharidin; then the mixture was administered intradermally
in the axillary region. Afterwards, the weekly dose of I-RNA
was 5 mg for the first 3 months; later, it was 5 mg every two
weeks. With the collaboration of the hospital and the
institute in a high-risk area, 21 patients began to receive
I-RNA treatment 2-4 weeks after their operations. The duration of I-RNA therapy ranged from 6-24 months, and the total
dose administered was 100-280 mg. Another group of patients
matched in age, sex, pathology and type of surgical resection
served as controls. These patients were treated with similar
routine medication without I-RNA.

The response to therapy was evaluated by the percentage
of survival. It was significantly higher within the first
fifteen months in the I-RNA treated group (86% as compared to
57%). This was especially obvious in the "minimum residual
disease" group (patients with blood AFP remaining above normal
after operation), and in early hepatoma (stage I) patients
(67% as compared to 11% in the control). No difference was
found among patients of "cured" group (whose blood AFP level
was back to normal after surgical resection). These patients
were followed up for two years. However, the long-term

percent survival at this time was found to be similar in both groups.[15] We are inclined to the view that I-RNA therapy may be useful for the very early hepatomas and subclinical hepatomas in combination with other therapeutic measures.

EXPERIMENTAL HEPATOMA RESEARCH

We have established a transplantable rat hepatoma, designated as BERH-2, by feeding Wister rats with diethylnitrosamine in drinking water. This hepatoma exhibited many fetal characteristics, including α-fetoprotein production, fetal isozyme expression (aldolase) and the presence of membrane-associated fetal antigen. We have also succeeded in establishing an in vitro cell line of this rat hepatoma. Using these model systems, as well as liver material derived from animals during DENA carcinogenesis and with regenerated and fetal livers, we have conducted our experimental hepatoma research work along the following two lines:

1) The expression and regulation of individual genes. Also, we have just finished the analysis of polysomal mRNA contents of AFP and ALB in BERH-2 hepatoma by studying their translational activity in wheat germ cell-free system. From the data shown in the tables 2 and 3, it is obvious that both AFP and ALB genes were stimulated in the hepatoma cells since more polysomal mRNAs were available in them as compared with normal liver cells.[16] We are now preparing the respective cDNA probes and attempting to clone these two genes in order to investigate further their activity and regulation.

TABLE 2

Comparison of Alb mRNA Level between Hepatoma & Liver

0.3ml Wheat Germ Incubation Vol.

PRNA 100ug	Total protein Incorp. cpm	Alb. Immuno-precipitate cpm	Alb/Total %
Exp.1			
Hepatoma	373980	1797	0.48
Liver	499260	1053	0.21
Exp.2			
Hepatoma	36180	595	1.10
Liver	89610	416	0.60
Exp.3			
Hepatoma	35656	545	1.52
Liver	33472	241	0.72

TABLE 3

Comparison of AFP mRNA Level between
Hepatoma & Liver

0.3ml Wheat Germ Incubation Vol.

PRNA 100ug	Total Protein Incorp cpm	AFP Immuno- precipitate cpm	AFP/Total %
Exp.1			
Hepatoma	373980	2067	0.54
Liver	499260	1013	0.20
Exp.2			
Hepatoma	24396	127	1.10
Liver	45809	183	0.40
Exp.3			
Hepatoma	360180	1044	2.40
Liver	89610	344	0.32

2) Studies of the changes of transcriptional activity
of the entire genome during DENA carcinogenesis and of BERH-2
hepatoma by the nucleic acid hybridization technique. So far,
only nonrepetitive and middle repetitive sequence transcripts
have been studied. The results indicated that transcription
of nonrepeated sequence DNA in BERH-2 hepatoma cell nuclei
was significantly higher than that in normal liver nuclei and
that the transcriptive products in hepatoma are mostly homologous to those present in fetal liver. On the other hand,
transcription of middle repeated sequence DNA was found to be
decreased in hepatoma cells. Furthermore, competitive inhibition experiments with the DNA-immobilized filter method showed
that the transport of RNA from nucleus to cytoplasm increased
gradually during DENA carcinogenesis (Tables 4,5 and Figs. 5,
6).[17,18,19] The significance of these findings, and their
relation to gene expression and regulation in hepatoma in
general, as well as to the expression of fetal characteristics
in particular, are still under investigation.
        This is a summary of what we have done and what we are
still doing in the field of liver carcinoma. In the future,
we will place particular emphasis on the oncodevelopmental
gene expressions in hepatoma cells and their relation to
cell differentiation and neoplasia in general.

FIGURE 5

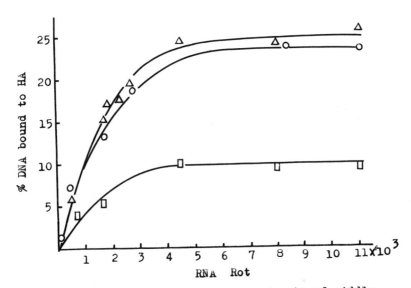

Saturation hybridization experiments of middle
repetitive sequence DNA and nuclear RNA
Reaction conditions: 0.12M PB, 60°C. Nuclear RNA
from BERH-2 hepatoma (□), rat embryonic liver
(O) and rat normal liver (Δ)

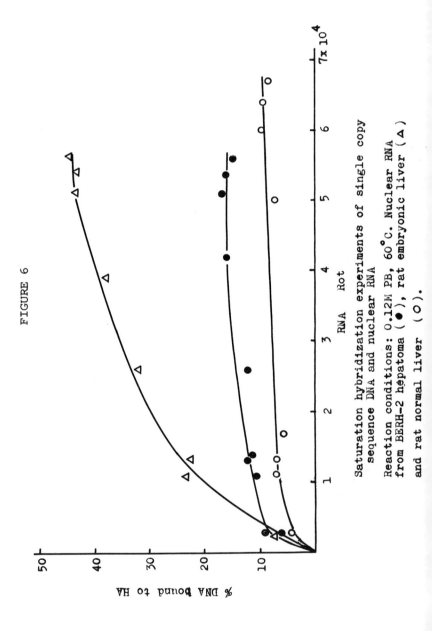

FIGURE 6

Saturation hybridization experiments of single copy sequence DNA and nuclear RNA

Reaction conditions: 0.12M PB, 60°C. Nuclear RNA from BERH-2 hépatoma (●), rat embryonic liver (△) and rat normal liver (○).

TABLE 4

Sequence organization of nuclear DNA
of rat liver and rat BERH-2 hepatoma

Nuclear DNA from	% Nonrepeated sequence DNA Cot > 200	% Middle repeated sequence DNA Cot 10^{-1} – 200	% Highly repeated sequence DNA Cot 10^{-1} – 10^{-2}
Rat liver	63.3 ± 3.3	26.0 ± 0.01	9.9 ± 0.6
Rat BERH-2 hepatoma	65.4 ± 1.1	24.2 ± 1.2	10.4 ± 2.3

Hydroxyapatite column elution assay method.

Reaction conditions: 0.12M phosphatebuffer pH6.8, 60°C

TABLE 5

Complexity estimation of nuclear RNA from rat liver, BERH-2 hepatoma and embryonic liver

	% of hybrids of nonrepeated sequence DNA with nuclear RNA from			% of hybrids of middle repeated sequence DNA with nuclear RNA from		
	liver	hepatoma	embryonic liver	liver	hepatoma	embryonic liver
Saturation value	9.5	16.0	44.0	25.0	10.0	23.5
% of total DNA complexity	12.4	20.8	57.2	12.5	5.0.	11.8
Complexity as kilobases	3.6×10^5	6.0×10^5	1.7×10^6	3.6×10^5	1.5×10^5	3.4×10^5

REFERENCES

1. Yao Zhen (1979) Basic research studies on liver carcinoma in China. *Zhonghua Zhongliu Zazhi (Chinese Journal of Oncology)* 1:230-232.
2. Chen Ruiming, Zhu Dehow, Ye Xiuzhen, Shen Dingwu and Lu Ronghua (1980) Establishment of three human liver carcinoma cell lines and some of their biological characteristics in vitro. *Scientia Sinica* 23:236-247.
3. Chen Hann-yuan, Chu Chih-mei and Tsung Hsiao-chien (1978) Studies on the karyotype and G-banding of chromosomes of human hepatoma cells. *Acta Biologiae Experimentalis Sinica* 11:171-182.
4. Raymond W. Ruddon ed. *Biological Markers of Neoplasia: Basic and Applied Aspects.* Elsevier, N.Y. (1978).
5. E. Boelsme and P. Rumke, eds. (1979) *Tumor Marker: Impact and Prospects.* Elsevier/North Holland Biomedical Press, Amsterdam, New York.
6. Abelev, G.I. (1971) Alpha-fetoprotein in ontogenesis and its association with malignant tumors. *Adv. Cancer Research* 14:295-358.
7. The coordinating group for the research on liver cancer, The People's Republic of China (1974). Alpha-fetoprotein assay in primary hepatocellular carcinoma, mass survey and follow-up studies. Presented at the 11th International Cancer Congress, Florence, Italy.
8. Shi Wei-kang, Lu Yan-ling, Ye Ming and Yao Zhen (1977) Membrane-associated embryonic antigen in human hepatocellular carcinoma cells. *Acta Zoologica Sinica* 23: 337-344.
9. Lu Yen-ling, Shi Wei-kang, Tieng Ling and Z. Yao (1978) Immunoelectromicroscopic study of membrane-associated fetal antigen on cultured human hepatoma cells. *Acta Biologiae Experimentalis Sinica* 11:73-77.
10. Tsung Hsiao-chien, Shi Wei-kang and Yao Zhen (1980) Immunoenzymatic localization of fetal antigen on human primary hepatomas. Paper submitted for publication.
11. Shi Wei-kang and Chen Zhen-kuo (1979). Extraction of surface antigens from human fetal liver cells with hypertonic potassium chloride. *Acta Biologiae Experimentalis Sinica* 12:169-172.
12. Pan Yu-Chih, Jin Shin-may and Sun Hsih-chum (1980) Cellular localization of surface and core antigen of hepatitis-B virus by immunoperoxidase technic. *Acta Biologiae Experimentalis Sinica* 13: in press.
13. Zhang Zong-liang, Wang Qui-da, Yang Song-yu and Wang Jue (1978) Microcytotoxicity assay of lymphocytes in hepatoma

patients against 5 $[^{125}I]$iodo-2'-deoxyuridine labeled human hepatoma target cells. *Kexue Tongbao 23*:185–188.

14. Yang Song-yu, Wang Qui-da, Chang Zong-liang, Ye Qinwei and Wang Jue (1978) Immune cytolysis of human liver cancer cells mediated by xenogenic "immune" RNA. *Acta Biologiae Experimentalis Sinica 11*:189–198.

15. Unpublished data.

16. Xu Yuen-chung, Liu Hai-hu, Xu Lian and Li Wen-yu (1980) Quantitation of mRNA levels of alpha-fetoprotein and albumin in transplantable rat hepatoma BERH-2. Submitted for publication.

17. Chang Yu-yen, Xu Yong-hua, Xu Ya-nan, Pen Su-fen and Lin Hui-wen (1978) Studies on the control mechanism of genetic transcription during rat liver carcinogenesis I. Comparative study of RNA complementary to the repeated DNA sequences. *Acta Biologiae Experimentalis Sinica 11*:97–104.

18. Xu Yong-hua, Peng Su-fen and Chang Yu-yen (1979) Changes of nuclear RNA and polysomal RNA complementary to the non-repeated DNA sequences in rat hepatoma. *Acta Biologiae Experimentalis Sinica 12*:237–246.

19. Unpublished data.

THE MECHANISMS OF ACTION OF CARCINOGENS AND TUMOR PROMOTERS AND THEIR RELEVANCE TO CANCER PREVENTION

I. BERNARD WEINSTEIN, M.D.
Division of Environmental Sciences
and
Cancer Center/Institute of Cancer Research
Columbia University
College of Physicians and Surgeons
New York, New York 10032

It is a great pleasure to participate with our colleagues from the People's Republic of China in this symposium on advances in cancer research. I had the privilege of recently visiting China and learning of the important work being done in cancer epidemiology and carcinogenesis. I am confident that through the increasing exchange of information between our two countries and the development of collaborative research programs, we can make great strides in cancer prevention. To do this, however, we will need a better understanding of fundamental mechanisms in carcinogenesis and improved methods for detecting potential carcinogens in our environment.

With respect to in vitro assays for carcinogens, we must consider several facts. 1) The uncertainty at the present time as to whether or not carcinogenesis results from simple random point mutations[1]. In the intact animal, and in humans, the carcinogenic process occurs via multiple steps that extend over an appreciable period of time[2]. Therefore, an ideal in vitro model system should display similar multiple steps and permit the analysis of each of these steps. 2) It appears likely that in the natural host carcinogenesis results from a complex interaction between multiple factors including electrophilic carcinogens, tumor promoters and hormones, various cofactors and, in some cases, interactions between chemical and viral agents[3,4]. Thus, in vitro bioassays should be available that have the capacity to assay for these diverse factors and for these multifactor interactions.

This research was supported by National Cancer Institute Grant CA-26056 and CA-21111.

In this paper I will briefly review the current status of in vitro transformation assays for carcinogens that act as initiating agents and then spend the rest of my talk discussing recent cell culture studies on the action of tumor promoters and on chemical-viral interactions.

SYSTEMS FOR STUDYING MALIGNANT CELL TRANSFORMATION IN VITRO

Table 1 lists the major in vitro systems in which chemical carcinogens induce cell transformation (for a detailed review see ref. 5). These include mainly fibroblast rodent cultures, either primary cultures or established cell lines. You will note that with most of these systems morphologic transformation does not occur until several weeks after carcinogen exposure. Although the hamster embryo system shows morphologic transformation within 7-10 days, a lag of several more weeks of serial passage is required for the full expression of growth in agar and tumorigenicity, a process termed "malignant transformation". The in vitro transformation by chemical carcinogens of epithelial cells and of human fibroblasts occurs with an extremely low frequency and a very long lag, even though these cells are not more resistant to the induction of specific mutations (i.e., to drug resistance) by chemical carcinogens. Thus, we see that the available examples of in vitro transformation already show aspects of a multistage process that is more complex than a simple point mutation. Data from several laboratories have indicated that the frequency of transformation of rodent cell cultures induced by radiation or carcinogens may be ten to several hundred times that obtained for the induction of mutations to specific markers such as drug resistance, even when both types of phenomena are scored in the same cell culture system[7-9]. This discrepancy is even greater when one considers the likelihood that cell transformation occurs via a multistep process which is limited, therefore, by the joint probabilities of each of the successive steps. This would suggest that the initial step induced by the carcinogen occurs with even a greater frequency than the net transformation frequency. Indeed, there is evidence that under certain conditions, i.e. the exposure of cells to chemical carcinogens[7,8] or radiation[9], at low cell densities, almost 100% of the originally exposed cells are capable of giving rise to progeny that are transformed. The fact that the phorbol ester tumor promoters can also enhance the transformation frequency in cultures previously exposed to chemical carcinogens or radiation[10-12], also provides evidence that we tend

TABLE 1

Examples of Cell Culture Systems That Can Be Transformed by Chemical Carcinogens

Type of System	Usual Endpoint	Scoring Time
A. Primary or Secondary Rodent Embryo Cultures		
1. Syrian Hamster	Morphological Transformation	8-10 days
2. Guinea Pig	Growth in Agar	4 months
3. Rat or Mouse Infected with Murine Leukemia Virus	Morphological Transformation	3-8 weeks
4. Rat Infected with Adenovirus	Morphological Transformation	25-40 days
5. Syrian Hamster Infected with Adenovirus	Morphological Transformation	25-30 days
B. Rodent Fibroblast Cell Lines		
1. 3T3 – mouse	Morphological Transformation	10-29 weeks
2. 10T½ – mouse	Morphological Transformation	4-6 weeks
3. BHK 21 – hamster	Growth in Agar	2-4 weeks
4. Rat Embryo	Morphological Transformation	40-43 days
C. Epithelial Cell Cultures		
1. Rat Liver	Growth in Agar, Cytologic Changes, Tumorigenesis	8-36 weeks
2. Mouse Epidermis	Growth in Agar, Morphological Alterations, Tumorigenesis	12-16 weeks
D. Human Skin Fibroblasts	Morphological Transformation	7-14 weeks

For further details and specific references see 5.

163

to underestimate the frequency of the initial event induced by chemical carcinogens or radiation. Some of the systems listed in Table 1 involve synergistic interactions between chemical agents and viruses and I will return to this aspect later.

Tumor promoters can be defined as compounds which lack significant carcinogenic activity when tested alone but markedly enhance the yield of tumors when applied after a low dose of an initiating carcinogen, for example benzo(a)pyrene (BP). The most potent tumor promoter on mouse skin is 12-0-tetradecanoyl-phorbol-13-acetate (TPA), and related phorbol diesters[14]. Elsewhere, we have contrasted the properties of initiating agents with those of the phorbol ester tumor promoters[1,15,16]. The major difference is that whereas initiating carcinogens usually generate electrophiles that bind covalently to cellular DNA (and are, therefore, mutagenic) this is not the case for tumor promoters. The two stage mouse skin carcinogenesis system has served as a paradigm for studies on the multistage aspects of carcinogenesis in several other tissues and species. Evidence that hepatocellular cancer, bladder cancer, colon cancer, and breast cancer also proceed via processes analogous to initiation and promotion has been reviewed elsewhere[3,14]. In addition, there are several recent studies indicating that the tumor promoting effect of the phorbol esters is not confined to mouse skin[16].

The cellular targets for the action of the phorbol ester tumor promoters are not known with certainty, but recent studies in cell culture systems have provided important clues. The effects can be classified into three categories (all of which conveniently begin with the letter "m"): mimicry of transformation, modulation of differentiation, and membrane effects (For recent reviews see 1,3,14,15,16).

MIMICRY OF TRANSFORMATION

TPA induces several properties in normal cells that mimic those often seen in transformed cells. This mimicry includes changes in cell morphology, growth properties, cell surface properties, induction of plasminogen activator (PA) and ornithine decarboxylase, increased prostaglandin synthesis, decreases in growth requirements for serum and Ca^{2+}, TPA induced loss of actin cables and TPA induced loss of metabolic cooperation (for review see refs. 3,14,16). TPA can enhance the stable transformation of fibroblast cultures previously exposed to a chemical carcinogen, uv or x-irradiation[10-12], an adenovirus[4,17], or Epstein-Barr virus[18]. As described below,

TPA can also induce the irreversible acquisition of anchorage-independent growth in "partially" transformed cells[19,20]. These stable or irreversible effects of TPA indicate that "initiated" cells have a qualitatively different response to TPA than normal cells.

Some of these effects, for example, the induction of ΓA[21] or the induction of cell adhesion[22] provide simple and rapid assays for the phorbol esters and related macrocyclic diterpenes. Detailed studies have shown a good structure-function relationship between these effects and tumor promoting activity on mouse skin[21,22], (Yamasaki, H., Weinstein, I.B. and Van Duuren, B., unpublished studies).

MODULATION OF DIFFERENTIATION

Since it is likely that carcinogenesis involves major disturbances in differentiation, it is of interest that TPA is a highly potent inhibitor or inducer of differentiation in a variety of cell systems (Table 2). The examples include a variety of programs of differentiation and cells from such diverse species as avian, rodent, human and even echinoderm. It is possible that the ability of TPA to either induce or inhibit differentiation depends on the nature of membrane constituents of the target cell. Reciprocal effects of the same agent on differentiation, depending on the target cells, have been seen with other agents including glucocorticoid hormones, cyclic AMP and BudR.

We have previously emphasized that the ability of tumor promoters to inhibit terminal differentiation may be an important clue to their action as tumor promoters on mouse skin[15,16]. The basal cells in the adult epidermis are continually dividing, yet the tissue is in a state of balanced growth. Presumably, this is because of asymmetric division of stem cells. One daughter cell remains a stem cell and the other daughter cell is committed to keratinize and terminally differentiate, thus, irreversibly losing its growth potential. If an "initiated" stem cell were restrained to this mode of division, it could not increase its proportion in the stem cell pool. If, however, the stem cell division mode was interrupted by the action of a promoting agent, the initiated cell could undergo exponential division thus yielding a clone of similar cells. Since TPA can also induce phenotypic changes in cells that mimic those of transformed cells, the microenvironment of a clone of such cells might itself enhance their further outgrowth and development into a tumor. In addition, clonal expansion of the population of

TABLE 2

TPA Modulation of Differentiation

Cell System	Type of Differentiation
Examples of Inhibition of Differentiation	
Chick Embryo Fibroblasts	Myogenesis
Chick Embryo Chondroblasts	Chondrogenesis
Chick Embryo Dorsal Root Ganglion	Neurite
Murine Erythroleukemia	Erythroid
Murine 3T3 Cell Line	Adipocytes
Murine Neuroblastoma	Neurite
Murine Melanoma	Melanogenesis
Hamster Epidermal Cultures	Keratinocytes
Mouse Epidermal Cultures	Keratinocytes
Rat Mammary Carcinoma	Dome Formation
Sea Urchin	Embryogenesis
Examples of Induction of Differentiation	
Murine Rauscher Virus Erythroleukemia	Erythroid
Human Myeloid Leukemia Cell Line	Macrophage and Granulocyte
Murine Myeloid Leukemia	Macrophage and Granulocyte
Human Melanoma Cell Line	Melanogenesis

For refs. see 3,14,16,33 and text.

initiated cells would provide a larger population from which variants that have undergone progression to later stages of neoplasia might emerge.

MEMBRANE EFFECTS AND PHOSPHOLIPID METABOLISM

There is considerable evidence that the cell surface membrane may be the initial and major target of TPA action[16]. Table 3 is a list of effects of TPA on cell surfaces and membranes. Several of these effects occur within minutes after exposing cell cultures to TPA and are not blocked by inhibitors of protein or RNA synthesis, suggesting that they result from a direct action of TPA on cell membranes. This is true for the enhancement of 2-deoxyglucose uptake, altered membrane "fluidity", altered cell adhesion, the induction of phospholipid turnover and the inhibition of EGF receptor binding. TPA induces an increase in the incorporation of P^{32} or choline into membrane phospholipids, deacylation of phospholipids and release of arachidonic acid, and increases prostaglandin synthesis[38-40].

Recently, R.A. Mufson in our laboratory has studied the release of choline metabolites from C3H10T½ cells prelabelled with (^{3}H) choline[29]. Within 5 minutes of exposure to TPA, the release of (^{3}H) choline metabolites was enhanced two-fold and by 60-120 minutes the release was 4-5 times that of vehicle controls. Choline metabolite release was concentration de-

TABLE 3

Effects of TPA on Cell Surfaces and Membranes in Cell Culture
Altered Na/K ATPase
Increased Uptake 2-DG, ^{32}P, ^{86}RB
Increased Membrane Lipid "Fluidity"
Increased Phospholipid Synthesis
Increased Release Arachidonic Acid, Prostaglandins, Choline
Altered Morphology and Cell-Cell Orientation
Altered Cell Adhesion
Increased Pinocytosis
Altered Fucose-Glycopeptides
Decreased LETS Protein
"Uncoupling" of β-Adrenergic Receptors
Inhibition of Binding of EGF to Receptors
Decrease in Acetylcholine Receptors
Synergistic Interaction with Growth Factors
Inhibition of Metabolic Cooperation

For refs. see 3,14,16,33 and text.

pendent between 10 and 100ng TPA/ml. Phorbol 12,13-dideca-
noate (PDD) was also active but 4αPDD, which is not a tumor
promoter, was inactive. The radioactivity released by TPA
was derived from phospholipids since changes in the acid soluble pool of choline metabolites were insufficient to account
for the amount of material released. The released material
was identified by chromatography as choline and phosphoryl
choline. Neither cycloheximide nor cordycepin blocked the
TPA induced release. The release was, however, temperature
dependent and did not occur at $4^{\circ}C$. TPA did not induce the
release of (^3H) inositol from prelabelled cells. We believe
that TPA induced choline release is due to activation of an
endogenous phospholipase C or D. This TPA effect is similar
to that of certain other agonists which also activate degradation of phospholipids, although in the previously described
examples the target is phosphatidylinositol rather than phos-
phatidylcholine[30,31]. It is not known how these membrane effects might induce signals or second messengers that mediate
the subsequent cytoplasmic and nuclear effects of TPA. An increase in intracellular Ca^{2+} concentration, enhanced protein
kinase activity, or release of yet unidentified mediators remain to be explored.

MEMBRANE RECEPTORS FOR EGF AND TPA

     TPA and EGF have similar but not identical effects on
cells in culture[32-35]. We discovered that TPA causes almost
an immediate inhibition of the binding of ^{125}I-EGF to cell
surface receptors and that it also causes a loss of previously
bound EGF from these receptors[45,47]. With a series of phorbol
compounds, or chemically related macrocyclic plant diterpenes,
this effect correlated quite well with the known potencies of
these compounds as tumor promoters on mouse skin. An exception is the compound mezerein which, although it is equipotent
to TPA with respect to several cell culture effects, and induction of ODC in mouse skin, is much weaker than TPA as a tumor promoter on mouse skin[36,37]. Recent studies suggest that
tumor promotion can be divided into two phases and that mezerein acts only during the second phase, whereas TPA is active
in both phases[37]. Studies with a variety of inhibitors[35,38],
suggest that the TPA inhibition of EGF-receptor binding does
not require RNA or protein synthesis, energy metabolism, or
cytoskeletal changes. Thus, the effect appears to be mediated
directly at the level of the plasma membrane. TPA inhibition
of EGF binding is not due to increased degradation of EGF or
increased internalization of the EGF-receptor complex[35]. The

effect of TPA on EGF receptors is an indirect one, perhaps related to TPA induced changes in the lipid microenvironment of the EGF receptors[35,38]. Our findings on TPA inhibition of EGF binding have been confirmed and extended by other investigators[41,42].

A curious finding is that with prolonged exposure cells become refractory to TPA-induced inhibition of EGF-receptor binding[47,50]. this is consistent with evidence that following prolonged exposure cells can escape from other effects of TPA[39,40]. This phenomenon could play an important role in tissue specific and dose-scheduling effects of TPA.

The ability of TPA to inhibit the binding of EGF to its receptors, to "uncouple" the β-adrenergic receptor and to cause a decrease in acetylcholine receptors in chick myoblasts (Table 3), suggest that the pleiotropic effects of TPA on cell growth, function and differentiation may relate, at least in part, to its effects on membrane receptors, thus altering the response of cells to extracellular signals. Possible affects on receptors involved in cell-cell contacts and TPA inhibition of metabolic cooperation[43,44] could also impair cell-cell recognition in TPA exposed tissues. It appears likely that TPA exerts such effects by binding to highly specific cell surface receptors (see below), and that this then leads to multiple changes in membrane structure and function. It is perhaps for this reason that certain membrane perturbing agents like the bee venom polypeptide melittin[45], and the Staph. aureus polypeptide delta hemolysin[46], can induce several effects similar to those of TPA. Thus our results with TPA may relate to the action of various drugs and toxins that have as their target the cell membrane.

We have previously postulated that TPA usurps the function of a cell surface receptor whose normal function is to mediate the action of a yet to be identified growth regulator or hormone[15,33]. The postulated endogenous factor that normally utilizes the receptor system usurped by TPA could play an important role in the control of stem cell proliferation and differentiation in various normal tissues. The fact that tumor cells can make polypeptide growth factors,[47,51] suggests that changes in the function of growth factor receptors may play an important role not only in the carcinogenic process but also in maintenance of the transformed state.

Blumberg's laboratory has recently employed ^{3}H-phorbol dibutyrate (PDBu) to obtain direct evidence that the membranes of fibroblast cultures and mouse epidermal cells do contain high affinity saturable receptors for PDBu, TPA and related tumor promoting phorbol esters[48]. We have confirmed and extended this finding and developed a simple assay for these re-

ceptors using intact monolayers of rat embryo fibroblasts[49].
Although TPA does inhibit the binding of ^{125}I-EGF to its cell
surface receptors, EGF does not inhibit the binding of [3]H-
PDBu to its receptors[33,48,49]. These results provide further
evidence that the receptors for the phorbol esters are dis-
tinct from those for EGF. Scatchard plots indicate that the
rat embryo cells contain about 2×10^5 high affinity PDBu receptors with a K_D of about 8nM[49]. The receptor assay for phorbol
esters should prove useful in further studies on the biochemical mechanisms of action of these agents and in the search
for the putative endogenous substance that normally utilizes
this class of receptors.

SYNERGISTIC INTERACTIONS BETWEEN CHEMICAL AGENTS AND VIRUSES
IN CELL TRANSFORMATION

There are several examples in which chemical and physical
agents interact synergistically with viruses in the carcinogenic process both in vitro and in vivo (for review see refs.
4,5,17). Indeed, it seems likely that certain human cancers
may be due to interactions between chemical agents and types
of viruses which alone would have little or no oncogenic potential. This is important to keep in mind in the search for
viruses that might play a role in human cancer causation.
These agents may not have all of the properties of oncogenic
viruses seen in experimental animal systems and, when assayed
alone, they may not be capable of cancer induction in the absence of chemical cofactors.
    To explore these aspects of chemical-viral interactions,
we have developed an in vitro system in which the transformation of rat embryo (RE) cells is markedly enhanced when, after
infection with a mutant (H5ts125) of human adenovirus type 5,
the cells are grown in the presence of TPA[17]. The presence
of TPA caused an increased number of foci of transformation.
Foci also appeared earlier and were larger than those obtained with adenovirus in the absence of TPA. Phorbol, 4αPDD,
and 4-0-MeTPA were inactive in this system. The addition of
TPA could be delayed until after viral uptake and integration
of adenovirus sequences into the host genome had occurred,
thus indicating that the enhancement by TPA was not exerted
on these steps.
    One of the best in vitro markers for the tumorigenicity
of transformed fibroblasts or epithelial rodent cells is anchorage independence, i.e., ability to grow in agar or agarose
suspension, although there are a few exceptions (for review
see 4,50). We have found that although TPA does not enhance

the growth in agar of normal RE cells, it does induce the
growth in agar of morphologically transformed adenovirus-
infected RE cells [19]. This effect appears to be inductive and
not due to simple cell selection. Yet it is irreversible,
since when the TPA is removed, the cells now grow in agar
with a higher efficiency than prior to exposure to TPA. Certain serially passaged mouse epidermal cell cultures also undergo an irreversible increase in anchorage-independent
growth when exposed to TPA[20]. This phenomenon may represent
a useful _in vitro_ model system for studying the process of tumor progression.

The synergistic interaction between initiating carcinogens and adenovirus was also studied in this system[17]. If
prior to infecting the cells with the virus, we exposed the
cells to benzo(a)pyrene or DMBA and then within 24 hours infected the cells with adenovirus, there was an enhancement of
cell transformation. These results, as well as those of
other investigators[52], suggest that, by damaging DNA and inducing DNA repair, initiating carcinogens increase the number of cells in a virus infected population that acquire sta-
bly integrated viral sequences[17,52,53]. The enhancement by
initiating carcinogens and by tumor promoters of adenovirus
transformation is additive, indicating that they occur by
different mechanisms.

It seems likely that these _in vitro_ interactions may be
relevant to the interaction between viruses, chemical carcinogens, tumor promoters, hormones and other cofactors in the
causation of specific human cancers, particularly liver cancer in Africa, nasopharyngeal carcinoma, Burkitt's lymphoma
and possibly breast cancer[3].

MOLECULAR MECHANISM OF INITIATION AND A UNIFIED THEORY OF
INITIATION AND PROMOTION

In the final analysis, the mechanism by which tumor
promoters enhance the conversion of initiated cells to
tumor cells must take into account the mechanism of
action of initiating carcinogens. Although current evidence
suggests that covalent binding of carcinogens like BP to cellular DNA is the critical event in initiation, the subsequent
biochemical events that lead to establishment of the initiated cell are not known. Several possible molecular mechanisms are listed in Table 4 and have been discussed in detail
elsewhere[1].

There has been a tendency to think of the initiating
event in chemical carcinogenesis as a simple random-point

TABLE 4

*Possible Molecular Mechanisms of Initiation of the Carcino-
genic Process*
A.   With Permanent Changes in DNA Sequence
  1.   Random point mutations
       a.   Direct: base substitution, frame shift or
            deletion in structural or regulatory gene.
       b.   Indirect: induction of "SOS-type" error
            prone DNA synthesis
  2.   Ordered gene rearrangements: transposition,
       amplification, deletion, etc.

B.   Without Permanent Changes in DNA Sequence
  1.   Altered chromatin structure, altered feedback loops,
       DNA methylation, etc.

For a more detailed discussion see ref. 1

mutation resulting from errors in replicating the damaged
DNA. However, certain aspects of the carcinogenic process
are not consistent with this simple mechanism[1-3]. In bacteria, physical and chemical agents that damage DNA, including chemical carcinogens, induce a highly pleiotropic response called "SOS functions"[54,55], which includes induction
of an error-prone DNA synthesis mechanism. Our laboratory
has recently found that mutagenesis by benzo(a)pyrene diol
epoxide (BPDE 1) in E. coli is mediated via this mechanism[56].
It is not known whether similar responses to DNA damage occur
in eukaryotic cells, and if so, what the components of this
response might be.
      Recent studies in both prokaryotic and eukaryotic cells
indicate that the linear arrangement of coding sequences in
DNA may be more complex and also more plastic than previously
envisioned[57-60]. It is possible, therefore, that highly
specific genome arrangements may be responsible for certain
aspects of development and differentiation in eukaryotic
systems, a hypothesis proposed by McClintock a number of
years ago[61]. It would not be surprising if chemical modification of the DNA by carcinogens disrupted these mechanisms.
One might further speculate that the "SOS" program of response to DNA damage in mammalian cells might result in
transposition of specific DNA sequences. By scrambling an
otherwise orderly process of genome rearrangements, carcinogens could produce distortions in cell commitment and thus
initiate the carcinogenic process. Phrased in other terms,

this theory postulates that during normal development, the establishment of specific populations of stem cells involves gene transpositions. By damaging DNA, initiating carcinogens induce aberrant forms of gene transposition, thus establishing aberrant stem cells. The subsequent role of tumor promoters might be to enhance the outgrowth of these cells (as discussed above), as well as "switch on" their aberrant programs of differentiation, just as normal growth factors might induce normal stem cells to express their specialized functions. Presumably, the phorbol ester tumor promoters accomplish this by binding to and usurping the function of receptors normally occupied by endogenous factors that control stem cell replication and differentiation. Following repeated exposure of initiated cells to TPA, a neoplastic population might eventually emerge which grows autonomously in the absence of TPA, perhaps due to further changes in genome structure. Several aspects of this hypothesis are currently being tested in our laboratory.

ACKNOWLEDMENTS

The author gratefully acknowledges the valuable contributions made to these studies by Drs. P.B. Fisher, A. Horowitz, J. Laskin, L.S. Lee, R.A. Mufson, and H. Yamasaki. He also thanks Evelyn Emeric and Patricia Vickman for valuable assistance in the preparation of this manuscript, and Janet Bozzone, Ester Okin and James Chi for their valuable technical assistance.

REFERENCES

1. Weinstein, I.B., Yamasaki, H., Wigler, M., Lee, L.S., Fisher, P.B., Jeffrey, A.M., and Grunberger, D.: Molecular and cellular events associated with the action of initiating carcinogens and tumor promoters. In: A.C. Griffin and R.C. Shaw, (eds.), *Carcinogens, Identification and Mechanisms of Action*, Raven Press, New York, pp. 399-418, 1979.
2. Foulds, L., (ed.), *Neoplastic Development, Vol. 1,* Academic Press, London and New York, 1969.
3. Weinstein, I.B.: Studies on the mechanism of action of tumor promoters and their relevance to mammary carcinogenesis. In: C.M. McGrath, M.J. Brennan and M.A. Rich, (eds.), *Cell Biology of Breast Cancer*, Academic Press, New York, 1980, in press.

4. Fisher, P.B., and Weinstein, I.B.: Chemical-viral inter-
    actions and multistep aspects of cell transformation.
    In: R. Montesano, H. Bartsch and L. Tomatis, (eds.),
    *Molecular and Cellular Aspects of Carcinogen Screening
    Tests,* IARC Scientific Publications No. 27, Lyon, France,
    pp. 113-131, 1980.
5. Fisher, P.B., and Weinstein, I.B.: In vitro screening
    tests for potential carcinogens. In: J.M. Sontag,
    (ed.), *Carcinogens in Industry and Environment,* Marcel
    Dekker Press, New York, in press, 1980.
6. Barrett, J.C., and Ts'o, P.O.P.: Evidence for the pro-
    gressive nature of neoplastic transformation. *Proc.
    Natl. Acad. Sci. (USA) 75:* 3761-3765, 1978.
7. Mondal, S., and Heidelberger, C.: In vitro malignant
    transformation by methylcholanthrene of the progeny of
    single cells derived from C3H mouse prostate. *Proc.
    Natl. Acad. Sci. (USA)`65:* 219-225, 1970.
8. Han, A., and Elkind, M.M.: Transformation of mouse C3H/
    10T½ cells by single and fractionated doses of x-rays and
    fission-spectrum neutrons. *Cancer Res. 39:* 123-130, 1979.
9. Kennedy, A.R., Fox, M., Murphy, G., and Little, J.B.:
    The relationship between x-ray exposure and malignant
    transformation in C3H/10T½ cells. *Proc. Natl. Acad.
    Sci. (USA),* in press, 1980.
10. Mondal, S., Brankow, D.W., and Heidelberger, C.: Two-
    stage chemical oncogenesis in cultures of C3H/10T½ cells.
    Cancer Res. 36: 2254-2260, 1976.
11. Kennedy, A., Mondal, S., Heidelberger, C., and Little,
    J.B.: Enhancement of x-radiation transformation by a
    phorbol ester using C3H/10T½ Cl 8 mouse embryo fibro-
    blasts. *Cancer Res. 38:* 439-443, 1978.
12. Mondal, S., and Heidelberger, C.: Transformation of
    C3H/10T½ Cl 8 mouse embryo fibroblasts by ultraviolet
    irradiation and a phorbol ester. *Nature 260:* 710-711,
    1976.
13. Berenblum, I.: Sequential aspects of chemical carcino-
    genesis: Skin. In: F.F. Becker,(ed.), *A Comprehensive
    Treatise,* Plenum Press, New York, pp. 323-344, 1975.
14. Slaga, T.J., Sivak, A., and Boutwell, R.K., (eds.),
    Mechanisms of Tumor Promotion and Cocarcinogenesis,
    Vol. 2, Raven Press, New York, 1978.
15. Weinstein, I.B., Wigler, M., and Pietropaolo, C.: The
    action of tumor promoting agents in cell culture. In:
    H.H. Hiatt, J.D. Watson and J.A. Winston, (eds.),
    *Origins of Human Cancer, Cold Spring Harbor Conferences
    on Cell Proliferation, IV,* Cold Spring Harbor Labs., Cold

Spring Harbor, New York, pp. 751-772, 1977.

16. Weinstein, I.B., Lee, L.S., Fisher, P.B., Mufson, A., and Yamasaki, H.: Action of phorbol esters in cell culture: Mimicry of transformation, altered differentiation and effects on cell membranes. *J. of Supramolecular Structure 12:* 195-208, 1979.

17. Fisher, P.B., Weinstein, I.B., Eisenberg, D., and Ginsberg, H.S.: Interactions between adenovirus, a tumor promoter and dimethylbenz(a)anthracene in the transformation of rat embryo cell cultures. *Proc. Natl. Acad. Sci. 75:* 2311-2314, 1978.

18. Yamamoto, N., and Zur Hausen, H.: Tumour promoter TPA enhances transformation of human leukocytes by Epstein-Barr virus. *Nature 280:* 244-245, 1979.

19. Fisher, P.B., Bozzone, J.H., and Weinstein, I.B.: Tumor promoters and epidermal growth factor stimulate anchorage-independent growth of adenovirus transformed rat embryo cells. *Cell 18:* 695-705, 1979.

20. Colburn, N.H., Former, B.F., Nelson, K.A., and Yuspa, S.H.: Tumor promoters induces anchorage independence irreversibly. *Nature 281:* 589-591, 1979.

21. Wigler, M., DeFeo, D., and Weinstein, I.B.: Induction of plasminogen activator in cultured cells by macrocyclic plant diterpene esters and other agents related to tumor promotion. *Cancer Res. 38:* 1434-1437, 1978.

22. Yamasaki, H., Weinstein, I.B., Fibach, E., Rifkind, R.A., and Marks, P.A.: Tumor promoter-induced adhesion of ds19 clone of murine erythroleukemia cells. *Cancer Res. 39:* 1989-1994, 1979.

23. Kinzel, V., Kreibich, G., Hecker, E., and Suss, R.: Stimulation of choline incorporation in cell cultures by phorbol derivatives and its correlation with their irritant and tumor promoting activity. *Cancer Res. 39:* 2743-2750, 1979.

24. Suss, R., Kreibich, G., and Kinzel, V.: Phorbol esters as a tool in cell research. *Europ. J. Cancer 8:* 299-304, 1972.

25. Wertz, P.W., and Muller, G.C.: Rapid stimulation of phospholipid metabolism by 12-0-tetradecanoyl phorbol 13-acetate and its specificity for tumor promotion. *Cancer Res. 28:* 2900-2904, 1978.

26. Levine, L., and Hassid, A.: Effects of phorbol-12-13-diesters on prostaglandin production and phospholipase activity in canine kidney (MDCK) cells. *Biochem. Biophys. Res. Commun. 79:* 477-483, 1977.

27. Mufson, R.A., DeFeo, D., and Weinstein, I.B.: Effects of phorbol ester tumor promoters on arachidonic acid

        metabolism in chick embryo fibroblasts. *Molecular Pharmacol. 16:* 569-578, 1979.

28.   Yamasaki, H., Mufson, R.A., and Weinstein, I.B.: Phorbol ester induced prostaglandin synthesis and [^{3}H]-TPA metabolism by TPA-resistant friend erythroleukemia cells. *Biochem. Biophys. Res. Commun. 89:* 1018-1025, 1979.

29.   Mufson, R.A., and Weinstein, I.B.: Phorbol ester tumor promoters stimulate rapid release of choline from cell phospholipids. *Proc. Am. Assoc. Cancer Res. (Abstracts) 21:* 117, 1980.

30.   Michell, R.H., Jafferji, S.S., and Jones, L.M.: The possible involvement of phosphatidylinositol breakdown in the mechanism of stimulus-response coupling at receptors which control cell-surface calcium gates. In: N.G. Bazaw, R.R. Brenner, and N.M. Giusto, *Function and Biosynthesis of Lipids, Proc. of the Int'l. Symp. Buenos Aires, Vol. 83,* Plenum Press, New York, pp. 447-464, 1977.

31.   Salmon, D.M., and Honeyman, T.W.: Proposed mechanism of cholinergic action in smooth muscle. *Nature 284:* 344-345, 1980.

32.   Lee, L.S., and Weinstein, I.B.: Epidermal growth factor, like tumor promoting phorbol esters, induces plasminogen activator in HeLa cells. *Nature 274:* 696-697, 1978.

33.   Lee, L.S., and Weinstein, I.B.: Tumor promoting phorbol esters inhibit binding of epidermal growth factor to cellular receptors. *Science 202:* 313-315, 1978.

34.   Dicker, P., and Rozengurt, E.: Stimulation of DNA synthesis by tumor promoter and pure mitogenic factors. *Nature 276:* 723-726, 1978.

35.   Lee, L.S., and Weinstein, I.B.: The mechanism of tumor promoter inhibition of cellular binding of epidermal growth factor. *Proc. Natl. Acad. Sci. (USA) 76:* 5168-5172, 1979.

36.   Mufson, R.A., Fischer, S.M., Verma, A.K., Gleason, G.L., Slaga, T.J., and Boutwell, R.K.: Effects of 12-0-tetradecanoyl-phorbol-13-acetate and mezerein on epidermal ornithine decarboxylase activity, isoproterenol-stimulated levels of cyclic adenosine 3':5'-monophosphate, and induction of mouse skin tumors in vivo. *Cancer Res. 39:* 4791-4795, 1979.

37.   Slaga, T.J., Fischer, S.M., Nelson, K., and Gleason, G.L.: Studies on the mechanism of skin tumor promotion: Evidence for several stages in tumor promotion. *Proc. Natl. Acad. Sci. (USA) 77:* 3659-3663, 1980.

38.   Lee, L.S., and Weinstein, I.B.: Studies on the mechanism by which a tumor promoter inhibits binding of epidermal growth factor to cellular receptors. *Carcinogenesis,*

in press, 1980.

39. Mufson, R.A., Fisher, P.B., and Weinstein, I.B.: Effect of phorbol ester tumor promoters on the expression of melanogenesis in B-16 melanoma cells. *Cancer Res. 39:* 3915-3919, 1979.

40. Diamond, L., O'Brien, T.G., and Rovera, G.: Inhibition of adipose conversion of 3T3 fibroblasts by tumour promoters. *Nature 269:* 247-248, 1977.

41. Brown, K.D., Dicker, P., and Rozengurt, E.: Inhibition of epidermal growth factor binding to surface receptors by tumor promoters. *Biochem. Biophys. Res. Commun. 86:* 1037-1043, 1979.

42. Shoyab, M., DeLarco, J.E., and Todaro, G.J.: Biological-ly active phorbol esters specifically alter affinity of epidermal growth factor membrane receptors. *Nature 279:* 387-391, 1979.

43. Murray, A.W., and Fitzgerald, D.J.: Tumor promoters in-hibit metabolic cooperation in cocultures of epidermal and 3T3 cells. *Biochem. Biophys. Res. Commun. 91:* 395-401, 1979.

44. Yotti, L.P., Chang, C.C., and Trosko, J.E.: Elimination of metabolic cooperation in Chinese hamster cells by a tumor promoter. *Science 206:* 1089-1091, 1979.

45. Mufson, R.A., Laskin, J.D., Fisher, P.B., and Weinstein, I.B.: Melittin, a bee venom polypeptide, shares certain cellular effects with phorbol ester tumor promoters. *Nature 280:* 72-74, 1979.

46. Umezawa, K., Weinstein, I.B., and Shaw, W.V.: Staphyl-ococcal delta-hemolysin inhibits cellular binding of epidermal growth factor and induces arachidonic acid release. *Biochem. Biophys. Res. Commun. 94:* 625-629, 1980.

47. Roberts, A.B., Lamb, L.C., Newton, D.L., Sporn, M.B., DeLarco, J.F., and Todaro, G.J.: Transforming growth factors: Isolation of polypeptides from virally and chemically transformed cells by acid ethanol extraction. *Proc. Natl. Acad. Sci. (USA) 77:* 3494-3498, 1980.

48. Delclos, K.B., Nagle, D.S., and Blumberg, P.D.: Specific binding of phorbol ester tumor promoters to mouse skin. *Cell 19:* 1025-1032, 1980.

49. Horowitz, A., Greenebaum, E., and Weinstein, I.B., un-published studies, 1980.

50. Montesano, R., Drevon, C., Kuroki, T., Saint Vincent, L., Handleman, S., Sanford, K.K., DeFeo, D., and Weinstein, I.B.: Tests for malignant transformation of liver cells in cultures: Cytology, growth in soft agar, and pro-duction of plasminogen activator. *J. of the Natl.*

Cancer Inst. 59: 1651-1658, 1977.

51. Fisher, P.B., Lee, L.S., and Weinstein, I.B.: Changes in epidermal growth factor receptors associated with adenovirus transformation, chemical carcinogen transformation and exposure to a phorbol ester tumor promoter. *Biochem. Biophys. Res. Commun. 93:* 1160-1166, 1980.

52. Casto, B.C., Pieczynski, W.J., and DiPaolo, J.A.: Enhancement of adenovirus transformation by pretreatment of hamster cells with carcinogenic polycyclic hydrocarbons. *Cancer Res. 33:* 819-824, 1973.

53. Fisher, P.B., Dorsch-Hasler, K., Weinstein, I.B., and Ginsberg, H.S.: Tumour promoters enhance anchorage-independent growth of adenovirus-transformed cells without altering the integration pattern of viral sequences. *Nature 281:* 591-594, 1979.

54. Witkin, E.M.: Ultraviolet mutagenesis and inducible DNA repair in <u>Escherichia</u> <u>coli</u>. *Bacteriol. Rev. 40:* 869-907, 1976.

55. Radman, M., Villani, G., Boiteux, S., Defais, M., and Caillet-Fauquet, P.: On the mechanism and genetic control of mutagenesis induced by carcinogenic mutagens. In: H.H. Hiatt, J.D. Watson and J.A. Winston, (eds.), *Origins of Human Cancer, Cold Spring Harbor Conferences on Cell Proliferation, Vol. 4,* Cold Spring Harbor Labs., Cold Spring Harbor, New York, pp. 903-922, 1977.

56. Ivanovic, V., and Weinstein, I.B.: Genetic factors in <u>Escherichia</u> <u>coli</u> that affect cell killing and mutagenesis induced by benzo(a)pyrene 7,8-dihydrodiol 9,10-oxide. *Cancer Res.,* in press, 1980.

57. Kamp, D., Kahmann, R., Zipser, D., Broker, T.R., and Chow, L.T.: Inversion of the DNA segment of phage Mu controls phage infectivity. *Nature 271:* 577-580, 1977.

58. Brack, C., and Tonegawa, S.: Variable and constant parts of the immunoglonlin light chain gene of a mouse myeloma cell are 1250 nontranslated boxes apart. *Proc. Natl. Acad. Sci. (USA) 74:* 5652-5656, 1977.

59. Herskowitz, I., Blair, L., Forbes, D., Hicks, J., Kassir, Y., Kushner, P., Rine, J., Sprague, G. Jr., and Strathern, J.: Control of cell type in the yeast Saccharomyces cerevisiae and a hypothesis for development in higher eukaryotes. In: W. Loomis and T. Leighton, (eds.), *The Molecular Genetics of Development,* Academic Press, New York, pp. 79-118, 1980.

60. Hoeijmakers, J.H.J., Frasch, A.C.C., Bernards, A., Borst, P., and Cross, G.A.M.: Novel expression-linked copies of the genes for variant genes in trypanosomes. *Nature 284:* 78-80, 1980.

61.   Finchman, J.R.S., and Sastry, G.R.K.: Controlling elements in maize. *Ann. Rev. Genetics 8:* 15-50, 1974.

SOME IMMUNOLOGICAL STUDIES
OF ESOPHAGEAL CANCER IN MAN

ZHANG YU HUI
Cancer Institute
Chinese Academy of Medical Sciences

Esophageal cancer is common in China. It is a big threat to the health and life of people particularly in north China. It has been one of the major research projects in the Cancer Institute of the Chinese Academy of Medical Sciences. This problem has been approached from different angles. In the Department of Immunology, my colleagues and I have been studying the general immune competence as well as the specific immune response against esophageal cancer in patients.

In the first part of my talk, I shall present data on nonspecific immunity.

1. Patients' lymphocytes were tested for PHA blastogenesis in vitro. 200 microliter of capillary blood obtained from ear lobe was cultured in the presence of PHA and blastogenesis was observed morphologically. Since this was done in high incidence area, it was impossible to use ^{3}H-TdR incorporation technique in the field station. We found that, in esophageal cancer patients, lymphocyte blastogenesis, as shown by the percentage of blastoid transformation, was decreased. This was more marked in patients with advanced disease, i.e., in clinical stage IV and with mediastinal lymph node metastases.

2. Macrophage is a cell type which actively participates in the host defence, but our knowledge about macrophage is mainly derived from animals. Not much is known about human macrophage. In our laboratory, human macrophages were harvested from skin blister induced by cantharidin (Figure 1). The cells shown here have morphology typical of macrophage. They are phagocytic. Using CRBC as targets, the phagocytic function of human macrophage was examined in vitro. It was shown that about 80% of the cancer patients studied, including that of the esophagus, showed depressed phagocytic activity (Table 1). After successful excision of the tumor, the phagocytic function usually returned to normal or nearly normal level (Table 2).

181

FIGURE 1

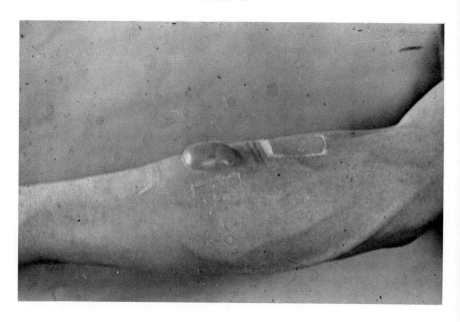

FIGURE 2

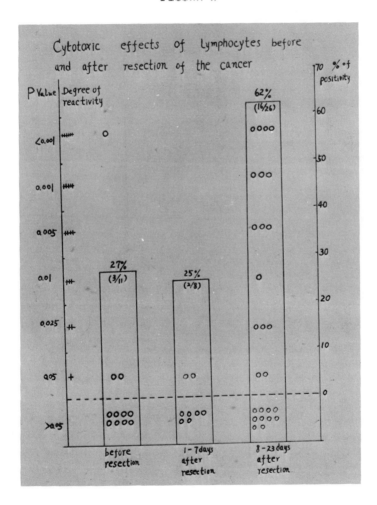

Cytotoxic effects of lymphocytes before and after resection of the cancer

TABLE 1

Phagocytic Activity of Human Macrophages

Subjects	No. of cases	Percentage Phagocytosis (%)	p
Normal	86	60.9±1.1	
Cancer patients recently diagnosed	167	40 3±1.1	<0.001
Cancer of esophagus and gastric cardia	33	37.8±2.4	"
Cancer of stomach	15	40.2±4.6	"
Cancer of colon and rectum	23	38.3±2.9	"
Cancer of cervix uteri	59	42.0±1.6	"
Cancer of breast	13	41.0±3.2	"
Other malignancies	24	40.9±3.2	"
Cancer patients survived for more than 3 years	83	56.3+2.7	>0.2
Benign diseases	54	65.5±1.8	<0.025

TABLE 2

PHAGOCYTIC ACTIVITY: 35 CANCER PATIENTS

BEFORE AND AFTER OPERATION

Test performed	Percentage phagocytels (Mean ± S.E.)	Phagocytic Index (Mean ± S.E.)
Before operation	36.80 ± 1.70	0.612 ± 0.057
After operation[*]	61.48 ± 2.61[*]	1.052 ± 0.065[*]

[*] P value less than 0.001 when compared with each other

3. Although phagocytosis is the major biological characteristic of macrophage, it may not be the sole form of defence mechanism for macrophage. Perhaps this is particularly true in the effector mechanism against cancer cell. It was shown that human macrophages were cytotoxic in vitro to cell line established from human esophageal cancer when the effector-to-target cell ration (E/T) was rather low. This macrophage-mediated cytotoxicity (MMC) was found to be nonspecific in nature. It could be observed in patients with esophageal cancer and in patients with other types of malignancy as well. These results were obtained using ^{3}H-TdR incorporation inhibition assay. However, the possible existence of thymidine in the culture medium as a normal secretory product of macrophage has made the results of this assay questionable. Macrophage-mediated cytotoxicity was also demonstrated on a visual basis by gross inspection and microphotography. With an increase in E/T ratio, more tumor cells were killed. Thus, this result makes the possibility that inhibition of ^{3}H-TdR incorporation is due to competition with cold thymidine rather remote. In order to quantitate MMC, the optic transmittance of wells was determined and it was found inversely proportional to the number of tumor cells inoculated. From the results so far obtained, MMC was observed not only in cancer patients but also in normal individuals. This gives a support to the immune surveillance theory in which macrophage might play an active part.

In the second part, I shall deal with the immune responses that are specific to esophageal cancer.

1. PBL isolated by gradient centrifugation on Ficoll-urographin from esophageal cancer patients were cytotoxic to esophageal cancer cells in vitro in 45% of the cases studied (Table 3). The positive rate and the degree of cytotoxicity were higher in patients who had their cancer removed (Fig.2).

2. The cell-mediated immune response was also tested by the leucocyte adherence inhibition assay (LAI). Using PBS extract of esophageal cancer as antigen, the adherence of leucocytes from the skin blister was inhibited in 67% of the patients examined. It is interesting to note that, among the 55 patients tested, 18 were very early cases and 11 of them gave positive LAI (Table 4). The cell-free exudate (CFE) abrogated LAI but this blocking effect was not tumor-specific. CFE obtained from cancer patients, either with or without tumor, all showed such an effect (Table 5). 25-30% of individuals who had different degrees of epithelial hyperplasia of the esophagus gave positive LAI (Table 6). This high false positive rate casts doubt on the specificity of the assay. But there may be alternative explanation. Since epithelial hyperplasia has been considered to be an

TABLE 3

Cell mediated cytotoxicity against esophageal and sarcoma target cells

target cells / patient groups	Eca 109	Ma
esophageal cancer	45% (21/47)	20% (8/40)
sarcoma	23% (3/13)	62% (13/21)
other cancer	18% (2/12)	18% (2/12)
normal	0% (0/23)	5% (1/21)

Eca 109 is an established esophageal cancer cell line

Ma is an established osteosarcoma cell line.

TABLE 4

LAI IN ESOPHAGEAL CANCER PATIENTS

PATIENT	NO. WITH POSIT. LAI/ NO. TESTED	PAI (%) (MEAN ± SE)
CANCER OF ESOPHAGUS	37/55 (67.2%)	44.37 ± 10.50
EARLY CASES	11/18 (61.1%)	42.71 ± 6.71
AFTER SURGERY	7/9	46.14 ± 8.37
SHORTLY AFTER INITIATION OF RADIOTHERAPY	7/10	47.78 ± 8.72

TABLE 5

BLOCKING OF LAI

PAI$_1$ (%)	CFE	NO. OF TEST	PAI$_2$ (%)	PB (%)
52.05	TUMOR-BEARER, AUTOLOGOUS	6	-7.43	112.78
	TUMOR-BEARER, HOMOLOGOUS	9	-7.83	128.78
47.25	TUMOR-FREE	5	-43.12	285.40

TABLE 6

LAI IN HYPERPLASIA OF ESOPHAGEAL EPITHELIUM

SUBJECT	NO. WITH POSIT. LAI/ NO. TESTED	PAI (%) (MEAN ± SE)
MARKED HYPERPLASIA	8/27 (29.6%)	-4.94±15.10
MODERATE HYPERPLASIA	6/24 (25%)	20.78±2.56
MILD HYPERPLASIA	6/19 (31.5%)	3.68± 5.81
NORMAL	2/7 (28.5%)	-4.91±11.77

important precancerous lesion and little, if any, qualitative
difference exists between marked hyperplasia and carcinoma
in situ, it is not impossible that they share some antigen
in common.

3. Patients were skin tested with autologous and homologous 3 M KCl extract of esophageal cancer for delayed-type
hypersensitivity (DTH). The test was usually performed 2-3
weeks after operation when they were positive to OT. Extract
of normal esophageal mucosa was used as control. Positive
skin reaction was obtained in 50% of patients when tested
with autologous tumor extract. Quite good correlation
between DTH and in vitro lymphocyte-mediated cytotoxicity was
observed. The positive rate was relatively low (36%) when
homologous extract was used.

The extracts of cancer and its normal counterpart were
purified by passing through Biogel P300 column. From the
eluate, two peaks were obtained. The first peak of the
cancer extract (C_1) (Fig. 3) was found to contain the active
component which elicited DTH.

4. Serum tumor-specific antibodies against esophageal
cancer were examined by the "single-well" cross-over electrophoresis which was devised by my colleague. In the conventional cross-over electrophoresis, two wells were used,
and antigen is added in one and antibody in the other.
During electrophoresis, antibody migrates toward the cathode
while the antigen toward the anode so that they form precipitate line at the place where they meet. However, antibody
does not always migrate toward the cathode. Some may migrate
to the opposite direction as well. If such is the case, it
is impossible for the antibody and antigen to meet. This is
probably one of the reasons for its low positivity. However,
in the single-well cross-over electrophoresis, antibody or
the serum sample to be tested, is put into the well and the
electrophoresis goes on. Then, antigen is introduced into
the same well and again electrophoresis continues but with an
opposite flow of current. At this time, antibody will
migrate back to meet the antigen. This device may provide a
better chance to capture the precipitate line. By single-
well electrophoresis, 5 lines were seen, 2 on the left and
3 on the right (Fig. 4). This indicates that some antigen
can also migrate toward the cathode. At the present moment,
this work has not gone too far yet but we found that the
precipitate line "a" might be specific for esophageal cancer
patients.

FIGURE 3

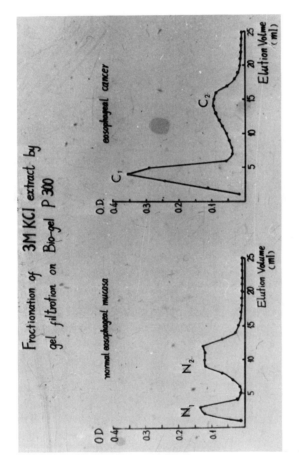

Fractionation of 3M KCl extract by gel filtration on Bio-gel P 300

FIGURE 4

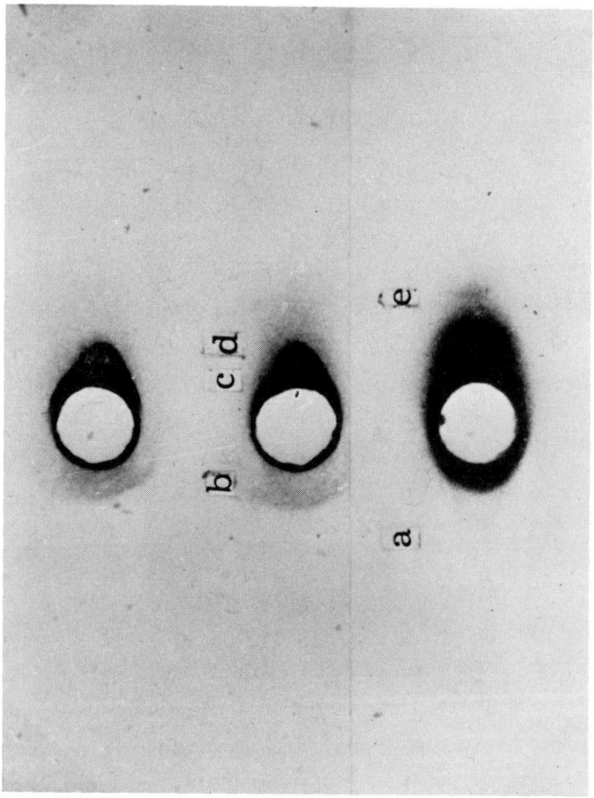

In summary, our studies indicate that the ability of lymphocytes to transform in vitro in the presence of mitogen and the ability of macrophage to phagocytose foreign particles are impaired in esophageal cancer patients. Their cytotoxic capacity is, however, less affected and can be demonstrated in vitro. Our studies also indicate that esophageal cancer probably has tumor-associated antigen which is immunogenic, i.e., the putative esophageal cancer-associated antigen can induce specific immune responses of the host, both cell-mediated and humoral. This encourages us to explore in-depth the potential of immunodiagnosis and immunotherapy of esophageal cancer.

NPC EPIDEMIOLOGY, RISK FACTORS
AND SCREENING FOR EARLY DETECTION

LI CHEN-CHUAN
Associate Professor,
Chungshan Medical College
Head, Clinical and Epidemiological Unit
of Cancer Institute
and
Head and Neck Department of Tumor Hospital

It is a great honor and pleasure for me to participate in this joint conference on cancer conducted by scientists from both the United States and the People's Republic of China, on the occasion of the fifth anniversary of the Julius and Armand Hammer Health Sciences Center and the Columbia University Cancer Center. I would like to express my heartfelt appreciation to the hosts of this conference for providing me with this opportunity. Through this conference, the friendship and cooperation between the scientists of our countries will surely be strengthened. As you all know, I am from the Kwangtung Province of China, which is a high area for NPC, and I would like to present some data about this. Because a wide range of contents are involved in NPC, I will focus only on some aspects of epidemiology, risk factors and screening for early detection of NPC.

A. EPIDEMIOLOGY

I. FREQUENCY OF NPC

Nasopharyngeal carcinoma (NPC) is very common in the Kwangtung Province of China. It represents 40.1% of all malignancies (41,004/102,329) (Table 1).[1] Among all malignancies of the head and neck NPC accounts for 85.2% showing a great predominance over the other cancers of the head and neck (Table 2).[1] Based on biopsy material from the entire Kwangtung Province, NPC accounts for 51.55% and one out of every two biopsied cancers in Kwangtung is NPC, among males, this ratio goes up to 66.70% (Table 3).[2]

TABLE 1

Percentage of several cancers among all malignancies
collected from Tumor Hospital of Chungshan Medical College,
Kwangtung Province, 1964-1979.

Site	Cases	%	Ranking
Nasopharynx	41004	40.1	1
Liver	16281	15.9	2
Lung	12893	12.6	3
Esophagus	7152	7.0	4
Cervix	6905	6.7	5
Breast	6643	6.5	6
Stomach	4400	4.3	7
Colon and Rectum	3855	3.8	8
Lymphoma	3196	3.1	9
Total (all cancers)	102,329	100.0	

TABLE 2

Percentage of several cancers among all malignancies of
head and neck collected from the Tumor Hospital of Chungshan
Medical College, 1964-1979.

Site	Cases	%	Ranking
NPC	41004	85.2	1
Larynx	1843	3.8	2
Thyroid	1617	3.3	3
Salivary gl.	1564	3.3	4
Tongue	1232	2.6	5
Maxillary sinus	887	1.8	6
Total (all cancers)	48,147	100.0	

TABLE 3

Percentage of several cancers among all malignancies based on biopsy material, Kwangtung Province, 1970-1972.

	Male		Female			Total	
Site	Cases	%	Cases	%	Unknown	Cases	%
Nasopharynx	6796	66.70	2478	31.56	9279		51.55
Cervix			2001	25.49	2001		11.11
Stomach	1356	13.30	504	6.41	1816		10.09
Breast	5	.00	1562	19.90	1567		8.70
Colon	780	7.65	605	7.70	1388		7.70
Skin	585	5.74	513	6.53	1098		6.10
Esophagus	383	3.76	91	1.16	474		2.63
Liver	289	2.85	98	1.25	381		2.12
Total (all cancers)	10,194	100.00	7852	100.10	18,004		100.00

II. *Prevalence Rate of NPC*

From 1970 to 1972, a mass survey of all types of cancer was conducted in several parts of Kwangtung Province of the total eligible 447,006 residents, aged 10 years or older, 436,786 (97.7%) were surveyed. The NPC prevalence rate was 39.84/per 100,000 pop., and age-adjusted prevalence rates were 58.6 for males and 22.8 for females (Table 4).[3]

TABLE 4

Prevalence rate of NPC for several parts of Kwangtung Province, 1970–1972

Site	Chugshan Co. (Pop. 242,757)		Lien-Chiang Co. (Pop. 83,273)		Chieh-Yang Co. (Pop. 51,635)		Total (Pop. 436,786)	
	No.of cases	Prevalence (per 100000)	No.of cases	Prevalence (per 100000)	No.of cases	Prevalence (per 100000)	No.of cases	Prevalence (per 100000)
Nasopharynx	133	54.8	14	16.8	12	23.2	174	39.8
All cancers	341	140.47	61	73.25	85	164.62	557	127.52

Different prevalence rates were noted in different parts of
Kwangtung Province: 54.8 for Chungshan County in the central
part of Kwangtung Province, 23.24 for Chiehyang County in the
eastern part and 16.81 for Lienchiang County in the western
part, showing an uneven geographic distribution of NPC (Fig.1).

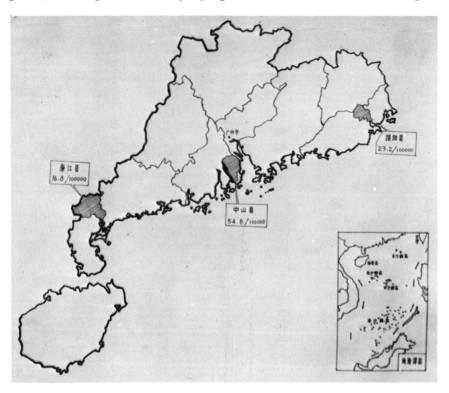

III. Incidence Rate of NPC

The incidence rate in Kwangtung Province was based on
biopsy material, 8.53 for males and 3.31 for females. The
data might be underestimated, because biopsies had not been
taken in a number of late cases (Table 5).[2]

TABLE 5

The incidence rate of NPC based on biopsy material of the whole province, 1970-1972.

Year	Incidence rate (per 100,000)		
	M	F	M+F
1970	7.95	3.14	5.54
1971	8.59	3.31	5.95
1972	9.04	3.47	6.25
Average	8.53	3.31	5.91

In 1970 a cancer registry was established in Chungshan County. The average incidence rates of NPC during the years of 1970-1975 was 21.59 for males and 8.66 for females (Table 6).[4] The curve shows no significant change of NPC incidence during the years 1970-1975 (Fig. 2), (Table 7).[5]

TABLE 6

NPC incidence in Chungshan County, 1970-1975.

Year	Incidence rate (per 100,000)		
	Male	Female	M+F
1970	19.86	8.69	14.28
1971	26.72	9.40	18.06
1972	20.61	8.96	14.79
1973	17.52	8.91	13.22
1974	22.40	7.55	14.98
1975	22.40	8.49	15.45
Average	21.59	8.66	15.13

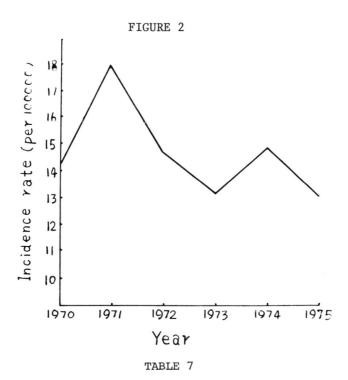

FIGURE 2

TABLE 7

Pathological classification of NPC in 7355 cases,
Kwangtung Province, 1970-1972.

Pathological type	No. of cases	%
Undifferentiated carcinoma		
Pleomorphic ca.	46	.62
Poorly differentiated carcinoma		
Squamous cell ca. grade III	3,761	51.14
Large round cell ca.	1,285	17.47
Fusiform cell ca.	176	2.39
Highly differentiated carcinoma	36	.49
Unclassified carcinoma	1,198	16.29
Nodal metastatic carcinoma	833	11.33
Lymphosarcoma	20	.27
Total	7,355	100.0

IV. *Mortality Rate of NPC and its Geographic Distribution*[4]

During the years 1970 to 1972, an intensive retrospective review of deaths due to NPC has been carried out in Kwangtung Province. NPC cases were found throughout the 107 counties and cities. The average mortality rate for NPC was 9.89 for males and 3.78 for females (Table 8).

TABLE 8

Average age-sex adjusted mortality rate for NPC in various districts of Kwangtung Province and the position of NPC among all malignancies.

Districts	Mortality rate (per 100000)		
	Male	Female	M + F
Shaoching	15.96	5.84	10.42
Foshan	14.21	5.67	9.71
Kwangchow	12.03	4.82	8.94
Hueiyang	10.62	3.82	6.24
Shaokuan	8.94	3.59	6.14
Chanjiang	7.49	3.06	5.37
Hainan	8.01	2.63	5.15
Swatow	6.13	2.59	4.31
Meihsien	5.62	1.96	3.44
Average	9.89	3.78	6.64

In Shaoching District, NPC mortality rate ranks first among all malignancies, with a mortality rate of 10.42, which is the highest among all the districts of Kwangtung Province. Meihsien District is the lowest, with a mortality rate of 3.44, which ranks fifth among all malignancies (Fig. 3).

FIGURE 3

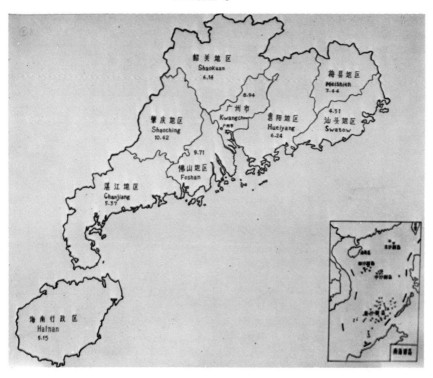

The results of analysis that was made according to the
four gradients of 3, >3, >6, and >9 per 100,000 pop. showed
that 21 out of 107 counties and cities in Kwangtung Province
had an NPC mortality rate of >9 (Table 9). Among these, 19
counties were located in the central part of Kwangtung
Province, including 9 in Shaoching District, 8 in Foshan
District and one in Kwangchow and Huiyang District, forming
a high-risk center of NPC with a mortality rate decreasing
toward its periphery. In the counties, the highest mortality
rate for NPC was 15.58, found in the Syhui County of
Shaoching District. The NPC high center is demonstrated in
Fig. 4.

TABLE 9

Counties and cities in Kwangtung Province with a NPC
mortality rate of > 9/100,000 pop.

Districts	County or City	Age-sex adjusted mortality rate (per 100000 pop.)
Shaoching	Syhui	15.85
	Deching	12.32
	Kwangning	11.94
	Fungkai	11.40
	Shaoching	10.08
	Loding	9.99
	Huaiji	9.53
	Sinsing	9.48
	Gouyao	9.38
Foshan	Chuhai	15.31
	Douman	12.32
	Penyu	12.14
	Foshan	11.69
	Chungshan	11.11
	Shunde	10.40
	Gouho	9.50
	Jiangmen	9.29
Kwangchow	Huahsian	12.35
Hueiyang	Tungkuan	9.33
Shaokuan	Liannan	10.16
	Shysing	9.24

FIGURE 4

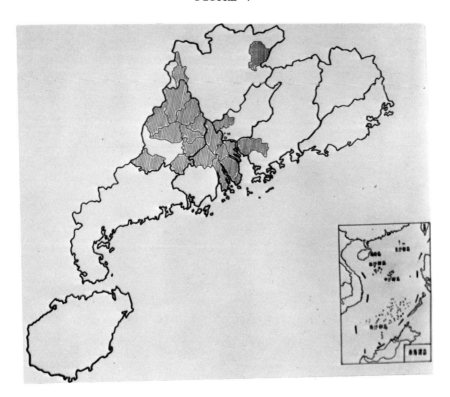

An important feature of the inhabitants living in the aforementioned NPC high-risk center is that most of them speak the Cantonese dialect. After their emigration elsewhere, they still maintained a much higher incidence rate of NPC than the local people.

"Boat" people, the earliest settlers in Kwangtung Province, whose NPC mortality rate (22.36) is the highest, are distributed over the delta of the Pearl River and also speak the Cantonese dialect. Through a long historical period, they intermarried with the Han people, and most of them now live ashore, while still retaining a much higher mortality rate of NPC than others.

Foodstuffs, water, rock and soil samples collected from various areas have been analysed with no definite relationship found.

The average mortality rate for NPC in Chungshan County from 1970 to 1975 was 12.46. This showed no significant

change from year to year, whereas that óf lung carcinoma
went up from 3.7 in 1970 to 8.3 in 1975, increasing two-fold
or more (Table 10), (Fig. 5).

TABLE 10

NPC mortality (per 100,000) in Chungshan County, 1970-1975.

Year	Mortality rate (per 100000)		
	Male	Female	M + F
1970	13.54	7.13	10.34
1971	16.56	8.31	12.44
1972	18.22	7.27	12.75
1973	17.74	6.58	12.16
1974	18.81	6.71	12.76
1975	19.97	8.70	14.34
Average	17.47	7.45	12.46

FIGURE 5

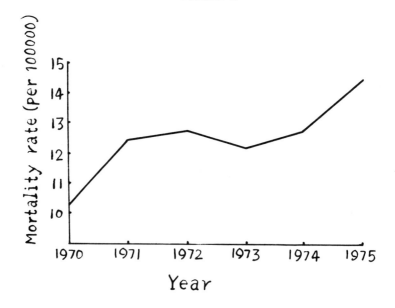

V. Age and Sex Distribution

The age-specific incidence rate for NPC of Kwangtung
Province represented by Chungshan County was 39.75 for males
and 14.59 for females, showing a higher incidence in males by
about three-fold (Table 11).

TABLE 11

*Incidence rate for NPC at various age groups in Chungshan
County, 1970-1975.*

Age Group	Incidence rate (per 100000)		
	Male	Female	M + F
10-	0.29	0.62	0.46
20-	7.30	3.20	5.25
30-	32.77	15.18	23.97
40-	68.02	29.90	48.96
50-	85.78	29.53	57.65
60-	66.69	22.21	44.45
70-	46.40	12.32	29.38
80-	10.71	3.72	7.21
Average	39.75	14.59	27.16

The curve of the age-specific incidence rate showed a
fairly steep rise after 20 years of age, with a definite
increase for each age group, reaching the peak between the
ages of 50 to 60, and then falling off after that (Fig. 6).

The curves for NPC in the Chinese population in Hong-
kong and Singapore are very similar with that of Kwangtungese
in Kwangtung Province. They show a fairly steep rise beginning at 20-24 years of age and continuing to about 50-54,
with a fall thereafter.[6]

It is of interest to note that in Tunisia and the
Sudan, the age curve appeared to be bimodal, 29% of cases in
the Sudan appearing before the age of 20 years.

The curve for NPC in Swedes is dissimilar insofar as
the rise occurs two decades later and continues until the
ages of 70-74.[6]

FIGURE 6

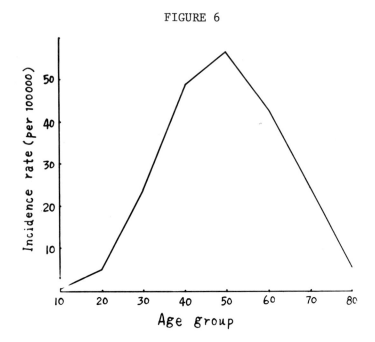

In Kwangtung Province, cases of NPC in children were rare. Among 16,536 cases of NPC seen at our hospital from 1964 to 1972, only 19 cases (0.11%) were children under 14 years of age, whereas in Liangning Province of Northeast China, a low-risk area for NPC, 41 cases (4.8%) out of 839 cases were under 14.[4]

The age-specific mortality rate for NPC in Kwangtung Province, represented by Chungshan County, was 37.03 for males, and 14.04 for females, also showing a higher incidence in males by about three-fold (Table 12).

The curve of age-specific mortality rate for NPC rises to about 60-70 years of age, with a fall thereafter (Fig. 7).

TABLE 12

Mortality rate for NPC at various age groups in Chungshan County, 1970-1975.

Age group	Mortality rate (per 100,000)		
	Male	Female	M + F
10-	0.29	0.15	.22
20-	2.51	1.80	2.15
30-	17.62	8.31	12.96
40-	54.56	20.32	37.44
50-	73.52	29.04	51.28
60-	79.41	27.22	53.31
70-	83.96	24.64	54.30
80-	21.42	14.88	18.15
Average	37.03	14.04	25.53

FIGURE 7

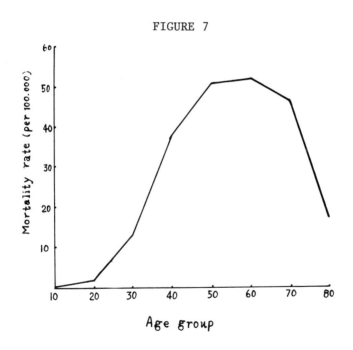

VI. Genetic Factors

Descriptive epidemiology has established that the population that speaks the Cantonese dialect has a high risk for
NPC, while those speaking the southern Fukien dialect (or
Teochow dialect) in Swatow District and those speaking Hakka
dialect in Meihsien District have a comparatively low risk
for NPC. This may reflect the different risk for NPC for
different population groups (Table 13).[4]

TABLE 13

*Age-adjusted mortality rates per 100000 per annum for NPC
among different dialect groups in Kwangtung Province.*

Kwangtungese dialect groups		Mortality rate (per 100000)
Cantonese	Chungshan County	12.46
	Boat dwellers	22.36
Southern Fukien	Swatow	4.31
Hakka	Meihsien	3.44

The incidence rates of NPC for both men and women who
speak Cantonese are twice those of the Teochow and Hakka
living in Singapore (Table 14).[7]

Familial aggregation of NPC takes place in both high-
risk and low-risk areas. From September 1979 to January 1980,
a total of 1000 newly diagnosed NPC cases (including 940
Kwangtungese cases and 60 cases from other provinces) were
found at OPD for NPC patients in our hospital. Among them,
100 NPC cases (10%) had a family history of cancer, including
110 relatives who had affected malignant tumors (Table 15).[8]
Most of the relatives belong to patients' sibs or parents
(Table 16).[8]

In Chungshan County, a case-control study of 244 NPC
cases showed that 10% of NPC cases had a history of occurrence of malignant tumors in other members of the family.
In 5% of these, the other tumors were also NPC. This was
most notable in sibs.[9]

TABLE 14

Age-adjusted incidence rates per 100000 per annum for NPC
among ethnic groups and in selected Chinese population

Geographical region	Males	Females	
Chungshan County	20.73	8.66	1970-1975
Hong Kong	24.3	10.2	Ho, 1972
Singapore			Shenmugaratnam, 1977
Chinese dialect groups			
Cantonese	29.1	11.0	
Teochow	18.3	6.2	
Hakka	12.6	4.8	
Fukien	14.1	4.7	
Hainanese	14.2	3.3	
Ethnic groups			
Chinese	18.7	7.1	
Malays	4.8	0.6	
Indians	0.9	0	
Japan	6.8	3.0	Sawak & Hirayama,1977
Hawaii	10.3	5.1	Waterhouse et al,1976
California	19.1	6.4	"

TABLE 15

Tumor types in 110 familial cases of 100 NPC cases with cancer family history

Types	NPC	Liver ca.	Lung ca.	Colon ca.	Breast ca.	Stomach ca.	Larynx ca.	Esophagus ca.	Cervix ca.	Others ca.
No. of cases	62	11	9	7	4	5	3	3	2	4
%	56.36	10	8.18	6.35	3.63	4.54	2.72	2.72	1.8	3.63

TABLE 16

Cancer frequencies in 110 relatives of 100 NPC cases with cancer family history

Pt's relatives	No. of cases	%
Parents	43	39.13
Sibs	38	34.54
Cousins	10	9.08
Aunts and Uncles	10	9.08
Grandparents	6	5.45
Sons and daughters	3	2.72
Total	110	100.00

NPC was highly prevalent in certain families. Among these, the Yeliang family was an outstanding example.[4] Among the 49 members of two generations of this family, there were 9 cases of NPC and one case of breast cancer (Figs. 8-11).

No significant change of NPC mortality on migration was found. Investigation revealed that the mortality rate of NPC for nonindigenous people (3.64) living in Canton City was much lower than that of the Kwangtung natives (10.90) living in the same area. The NPC mortality rate of Kwangtung people (7.10) living in Shanghai was found to be markedly higher than that of the local people (2.7). After their emigration to Shanghai, Kwangtung people still maintained a much higher incidence rate for NPC than the local people.[4]

FIGURE 8

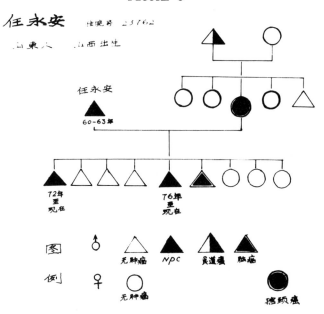

FIGURE 9

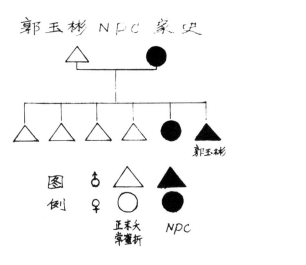

214

FIGURE 10

叶 X 一家族史調查图

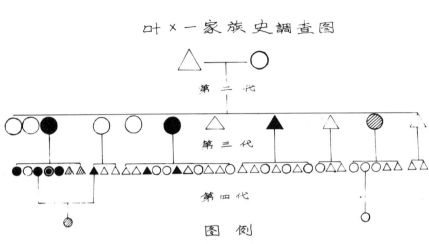

第 二 代

第 三 代

第 四 代

图 例

正未天
常查折 NPC NPC? 乳癌

FIGURE 11

梁 X NPC 家史

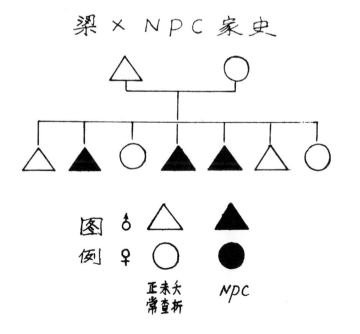

图
例

正未天
常查折 NPC

215

VII. Occupation

Most of the patients we investigated were peasants (55.56%) and workers (20.52%), who lived at a comparatively low economic level.[10]

"Boat" people who had the highest mortality rate for NPC (22.36) were largely fishermen or engaged in transportation. However, fishermen elsewhere do not have a high risk for NPC.

VIII. Environmental Factors

A retrospective case-control study of 304 NPC cases seen at the Tumor Hospital and 238 controls (noncancerous patients) from Ophthalmology and Surgical Clinics was conducted in 1964-1965.[11] In 1970-1972 a second case-control study of 244 NPC cases and matched controls was conducted in Chungshan County.[9] Also, an interview of 1000 NPC cases was conducted in OPD for NPC patients in the Tumor Hospital in September 1979-January 1980. No risk factor for NPC other than family history of disease was discovered.

A search for trace elements in food and drinking water has been taken. We tried to correlate levels of these metals with NPC mortality rate, but found that only the nickel levels in rice had any significant positive correlation with NPC mortality. A similar positive correlation was found between nickel levels in drinking water and NPC mortality rates. However, nickel levels in drinking water did not correlate with mortality rates for cancers of seven other sites (liver, stomach, esophagus, intestine, lung, breast, and uterus).[4]

800 pigs were surveyed, and 23 were found with nasal symptoms. In autopsies of the heads, 12 were found to have carcinoma. Two of these were squamous cell carcinoma of the nasopharynx, and the other ten were carcinomas of the nasal cavity and maxillary sinus. The remaining 11 pigs had inflammatory changes in the nasal cavity and nasopharynx, including heterophasia and atypical hyperplasia.[4]

B. EBV SEROLOGY[12]

Recently, sera from NPC patients, and other malignant tumor patients and healthy controls from 7 provinces and Beijing, were tested for EB-VCA-IgA antibody by immunofluorescence test. As shown in Table 17, 90.14% of 781 untreated NPC patients had EB-VCA-IgA antibody with a GMT of 1:15.32, whereas a very low frequency with a low level of

TABLE 17

A comparison of positivity and GMT of VCA-IgA
for patients of NPC, other malignant tumors, and normal individuals

	NPC pts Pretreatment	Other malignant tumors of H and N	Other malignancies	Normal individuals
No. of cases	781	91	268	171
No., Positive	704	3	7	–
%, Positive	90.14	3.30	2.61	–
GMT	15.32	1.32	1.30	1.25

TABLE 18

Comparison of positivity and GMT of VCA-IgA to EBV

for sera of NPC patients in 8 provinces (or city) in China

	Beijing	Kwangtung	Kwangsi	Fukien	Hunan	Yunan	Kiangsi	Kweichow	Total
No. of cases	165	131	320	32	55	18	23	37	781
No. positive	144	118	301	28	55	14	21	33	704
% positive	87.27	90.08	94.06	87.50	100	77.78	91.30	89.19	90.14
GMT	15.41	15.60	14.99	10.22	25.11	10.40	13.93	14.82	15.32

GMT of EB-VCA-IgA antibody was found in other cancers of the
head and neck or elsewhere, and no such antibody was found in
healthy controls.

There was no marked difference in the frequency and GMT
of EB-VCA-IgA antibody among NPC patients from different areas
in China (Table 18).

The frequency and GMT of EB-VCA-IgA antibody were
similar in 638 untreated NPC patients from Stage I-IV.   In
stage I NPC patients, whose tumor burden was minimal and
localized within one wall of nasopharynx, there was already
a very high level of EB-VCA-IgA antibody.   Therefore, the
detection of VCA-IgA antibody is valuable in diagnosis for
NPC, especially in its early stage or in patients with no
visible primary tumor mass in nasopharynx (To), but with
cervical lymphadenopathy (Table 19).

TABLE 19

*Relationship between VCA-IgA antibodies and clinical stages
for NPC patients*

Staging	No. of cases	No. positive	% positive	GMT
I	31	29	93.55	10.00
I	208	183	87.98	13.23
III	281	225	80.07	16.91
IV	118	109	92.37	17.47
Total	638	546	85.58	15.31

The level of VCA-IgA declined gradually with an increase
in survival duration after radiotherapy among 1711 NPC
patients.   When recurrence or distant metastasis occurred,
the VCA-IgA antibody increased again and reached its
original level (Table 20).

TABLE 20

Comparison of VCA-IgA antibodies and the length
of duration after radio-therapy for NPC patients

	Pretreatment	During radiation	<1 yr. after radiation	1-4 yrs. after radiation	4-22 yrs. after radiation	recurrence or distant metastasis
No. of cases	781	371	289	102	56	112
No. positive	704	315	224	62	22	96
% positive	90.14	84.91	77.51	60.78	39.29	85.71
GMT	15.32	9.12	9.81	5.65	3.12	15.52

A longitudinal follow-up of NPC patients showed that VCA-IgA antibody titres could be used as a warning signal for recurrence prior to clinical evidence. This brought further evidence of the strong association between EBV and NPC, and also suggested the possibility that EBV serology could be used by clinicians as a marker for prognosis after radio-therapy and for management of the treatment of the disease.

C. SCREENING FOR EARLY DETECTION

I. *General population screening for NPC:*

In a mass survey, conducted during 1970-1975, of 436,786 residents by nasopharyngoscopy, 174 NPC cases, including 80 newly discovered cases, were diagnosed (Table 21). Among those newly discovered cases, 43 cases (53.75%) were in stage I, while stage I NPC patients seen at the OPD for NPC patients in the Tumor Hospital from September 1979 to January 1980 comprised only 6%. Therefore, stage I NPC patients in the Mass Survey Group is 7.96 times higher than thos of the Hospital Group (Table 22).[3]

TABLE 21

Prevalence rate for all malignancies and NPC
as determined by a mass survey in several parts of Kwangtung Province, 1970-1972

Site	Male		Female		M + F	
	No. of cases	Prevalence (per 100000 pop.)	No. of cases	Prevalence (per 100000 pop.)	No. of cases	Prevalence (per 100000 pop.)
NPC	122	53.49	52	24.91	174	39.84
All malignancies	277	121.46	280	134.40	557	127.52

TABLE 22

A comparison of clinical stages of NPC patients between mass surveyed cases and hospital cases.

Stage	Mass surveyed cases		Hospital cases	
	No.	%	No.	%
I	43	53.75	56	6.0
II	27	33.75	406	43.2
III	8	10.00	302	32.1
IV	2	2.50	176	18.7
Total	80	100.00	940	100.0

In Chungshan County, such surveys were conducted by barefoot doctors trained to use postnasal mirror. The percentage of stage I and II NPC cases rose from 44.93% in 1970, to 68.86% in 1975, since the anticancer network was set up.

In Changshan County, 242,757 residents were examined by nasopharyngoscopy. Among them, 555 cases (228.6 per 100,000 pop.) of hyperplastic mucosal lesions were found, in whom 33 NPC cases in stage I were confirmed by pathological examination. These hyperplastic mucosal lesions might be represented premalignant changes of NPC.

II. Serological Survey[13]

Sera from 56,584 residents of over 30 years of age in 6 communes of Tsanzwu County (another high-risk area for NPC in Kwangsi Chang Autonomous Region) were tested for EB-VCA-IgA antibody by immunoenzymic method; 117 (206.8 per 100,000 pop.) had VCA-IgA antibody with a GMT of 1:21.1. Among these 117 persons, 18 were later diagnosed as NPC by clinical and pathological examination. 7 cases were in stage I, 4 were in stage II, 5 in stage III and 2 in stage IV (Table 23).

In 1979, sera from 136 patients with hyperplastic mucosal lesions of nasopharynx were taken for testing VCA-IgA antibody by immunoenzymic method; 27 persons had positive results and 4 of them were confirmed as NPC by pathological examination (Table 24).

TABLE 23

Results of serological survey for early detection of NPC patients.

Positive sera			NPC confirmed				
				Clinical stage			
No. of cases	No. of positives	GMT	No. of cases	I	II	III	IV
56,584	117	1:21.1	18	7	4	5	2

TABLE 24

VCA-IgA Detection for patients with hyperplastic mucosal lesion of nasopharynx

No. of sera	No. of positive sera	No. of NPC cases confirmed
136	27	4

D. PATHOLOGICAL CLASSIFICATION[10]

The vast majority of NPC arises from the nasopharyngeal epithelium and should be considered, irrespective of their appearance on light microscopy, as variants of squamous cell carcinoma. The pathological classification of NPC in 7725 cases collected from the Tumor Hospital of Chungshan Medical College (1970-1972) were distributed as follows (Table 25): undifferentiated carcinoma (or pleomorphic carcinoma) accounts for 5.38%; poorly differentiated carcinoma, 67.58%, including squamous cell carcinoma, Grade III, 48.68%; large round cell carcinoma (or vesicular nuclear carcinoma, or so-called lymphoepithelioma), 16.63%; and fusiform cell carcinoma, 2.27%; highly differentiated carcinoma (squamous cell carcinoma, Grades I and II), 0.47%.

TABLE 25

Percentage of NPC and head and neck cancers among all malignancies collected from the Tumor Hospital of Chungshan Medical College, Kwangtung Province, 1964-1979.

Site	No. of cases	%
NPC	41004	31.5
H and N	52485	40.4
All malignancies	130024	100.0

E. PATTERNS OF HOST RESPONSE (CLINICAL CHARACTERISTICS)

I. Clinical courses of NPC:

The clinical course of NPC varies widely in duration; without any form of specific therapy, the patients may live from 3 to 69 months, with an average of 18.7 months. As for patients in late stages, it ranges from 1 to 31 months, with an average of 7.9 months.[14]
The presenting symptoms depend on the location within the nasopharynx of the primary tumor, its tendency to invade neighboring structures, the direction of invasion, and its predilection to metastasize to regional lymph nodes. Thus, the signs and symptoms, in order of frequency, are cervical nodal enlargement, nasal symptoms (obstruction, postnasal bloody discharge, epistaxis), aural symptoms due to Eustachian tubal obstruction (impairment of hearing of the conductive type, with or without tinnitus and serous otitis media), persistent headache and involvement of cranial nerves (V, especially its mandibular branch, VI, IX, XII, etc.) (Table 26)[15]

TABLE 26

Order of frequencies of symptoms and signs in NPC patients: all cases (1000)

Presenting symptoms*	Frequency	%
Cervical nodal enlargement	774	77.4
Nasal bloody discharge and epistaxis	737	73.7
Nasal obstruction	480	48.0
Tinitus	626	62.6
Impairment of hearing	499	49.9
Headache	686	68.6
Cranial nerve involvement	451	45.1

* 127 cases (12.7%) have not any nasal or aural symptoms and signs, but only presented with cervical nodal enlargement.

II. Clinical Types of Disease[15,16]

The biological behavior of the tumor determines the clinical types of the disease. Since 1958, we have noticed that some cases of NPC with advanced cervical lymph node metastasis show total absence of involvement of cranial nerves, while others with marked lesions of the cranial nerves show no enlargement of the cervical lymph node. Still others have lesions in both sides. This led us to the question of whether the tumor, once it extended beyond its original site, would assume a definite or fixed pattern of evolution. This was found to be so in our study of 1,723 late cases (stage III and IV) drawn from 2,000 cases attended from 1960 through February 1966. Our findings were as follows:

1. The Cranial Type (A or Ascending Type): The cranial type, constituting about 10.91% of all late cases, is characterized by direct extension of the tumor toward the base of the skull with involvement of the cranial nerves II, III, IV, V, VI and/or destruction of the bone, but without cervical lymphadenopathy and distant metastasis, even up until the death of the patient. However, in a few patients, haematogenous metastasis may occur. Presumably, these metastases are the result of tumor invasion of the basal venous sinuses, which communicate with the internal jugular vein and perivertebral plexus of veins.

2. Generalized Cervical Lymphadenopathy Type (D or

Decending Type): The descending type occurs in about 35.98%
of all late cases and has the special feature of extensive
metastases in the cervical lymph nodes on one or both sides,
with a large mass of more than 8 x 8 cm. The lymph nodes
from below the clavicle to as low as the inguinal nodes and
retroperitionial lymph nodes, etc., may be involved. This
type is prone to blood-borne metastases, especially when the
supraclavicular lymph nodes are involved or the metastatic
mass reached the size of >8 x 8 cm. But this type did not
affect the cranial nerves II, III, IV, V^1 and VI.

3. Mixed Type (AD or Ascending-Descending Type): The
mixed type, constituting about 22.11%, is characterized by a
combination of the direct spread of the primary tumor and the
appearance of cervical nodal metastases. However, cervical
lymphadenopathy usually remains localized for a long time and
the size of the mass rarely reaches 8 x 8 cm.

On the basis of the analytic data in Table 27, the clinical type of stages I and II cases may be predicted. As shown
in Table 28, when a patient has a headache as the first symp-
tom and also has aural and/or nasal complaints but no cervical
lymphadenopathy, it may be presumed that the chance of the
case developing naturally into Type A is much greater than
its developing into Type D or AD, especially if the pathologic
diagnosis should be fusiform cell carcinoma. We feel that
this method, uncertain as it may be, still has some practical
bearing on prognosis and radiation treatment (to determine
the radiation dosage in nasopharyngeal or cervical region
according to the Type predicted). But a study of a large
series must be made before any definite conclusions can be
drawn.

III. Treatment and Prognosis

NPC is sensitive both to radiation and to many chemical
drugs. Radiotherapy constitutes the major form of treatment,
combined with chemotherapy before or after radiotherapy.
Out of 34,471 cases diagnosed by the Tumor Hospital of
Chungshan Medical college from 1964 to 1977, 16,645 cases
(47.91%) had been treated by irradiation with split course
treatment. 15,629 cases (93.9%) were followed-up until
February 1979. There were five- and ten-year survival rates
for, respectively, 31.27% (2947/9423) and 21.69% (781/3601)
(Table 29) [17].

TABLE 27

Comparison of important symptoms and signs
and pathological types in A, D, and AD types

Clinical types	Headache as 1st symptom (%)	Naso-aural symptoms (%)	Cervical adenopathy as 1st symptom (%)	Distant metastasis	Pathological types (in order of frequency)
A	54.3	98.9	0	–	Squamous cell ca. Grade III Pleomorphic cell ca. Fusiform cell ca. Large round cell ca. (rare)
D	14.6	78.2	69.8	+++	Squam. cell ca. Grade III Large round cell ca. and Pleomorphic cell ca. (very often) Fusiform cell ca. (few)
AD	31.7	98.2	49.6	++	Squam. cell ca. Grade III (most) Pleomorphic cell ca. Fusiform cell ca. Large round cell ca. (few)

TABLE 28

Prediction of clinical type in stage and cases of NPC

Headache as 1st symptom	Naso-aural symptoms	Cervical adenopathy as 1st symptom	Pathological type	Predicted clinical type
+	+	–	Fusiform cell ca.	A
–	+* –	+	Large round cell ca.	D
+	+	+	All types but large round cell ca. rarer	AD

* Either absent or mild

229

TABLE 29

Radiation treatment and prognosis of 16645 NPC cases
in the Tumor Hospital of Chungshan Medical College, 1964-1977

	Total	Treated	Follow-up	5 year survival	10 year survival
No. of cases	34,741	16,645	15,629	2947/9423	781/3601
%	100	47.91	93.9	21.27	21.69

Forty-five cases of NPC have occurred second or third primary cancer in 17,394 cases of NPC patients at the post-irradiation period. Most of them (25 cases) were located in the head and neck region, with 11 cases of squamous cell carcinoma of the tongue, which may have been due to radiogenic (Table 30)[18].

TABLE 30

Occurrence of 2nd and 3rd primary cancer in 17,394 cases of NPC patients at postradiation period, 1964-1978.

Site of 2nd or 3rd primary ca.	No. of cases	
H and N	25	
Tongue ca.		11
Thyroid ca.		3
Skin ca.		2
Larynx ca.		1
Maxillary ca.		1
Malignant mixed tumor of maxillary sinus		1
Fibrosarcoma of upper jaw		1
Fibrosarcoma of upper gum		1
Osteogenic sarcoma of lower jaw		1
Neurofibrosarcoma of supraclavicular fossa		1
Fibrosarcoma of external meatus		1
Fibrosarcoma of temperal region		1
Other sites	20	
Rectum ca.		5
Stomach ca.		3
Breast ca.		3
Corpus uteri ca.		3
Cervix ca.		2
Esophagus ca.		1
Penis ca.		1
Ovary ca.		1
Leukemia		1
Total	45	

REFERENCES

1. Data of the Tumor Hospital, Chungshan Medical College,
    Canton, China, 1964-1979.
2. Coordinating Group of Chungshan Medical College for NPC:
    *New Medicine (Canton):5(7)*310, 1974.
3. Tumor Hospital of Chungshan Medical College: *Research
    for Prevention and Treatment for Cancer (Beijing)(1)*:
    1, 1973.
4. Coordinating Group for Research on NPC: A Preliminary
    Investigation on the Epidemiology of NPC in Four
    Provinces and One Autonomous Region of South China,
    presented at 12th International Cancer Congress,
    Buenos Aires, 1978.
5. Data of Tumor Prevention Team, Chungshan County Hospital.
6. Gude-The, et al: Nasopharyngeal Carcinoma, in: A.S.
    Evans (Ed.), *Viral Infections of Humans*, 1976.
7. K. Sharmugaratnam: Variations in NPC Incidence Among
    Specific Chinese Communities (Dialect Groups) in
    Singapore, in: *NPC: Etiology and Control*, IARC, 1978.
8. Data of OPD for NPC in the Tumor Hospital of Chungshan
    Medical College, 1979.
9. Tumor Prevention Team of Tumor Hospital of Chungshan
    Medical College, *New Medicine (Canton):12*: 15, 1972.
10. Coordinating Group of Kwangtung Province for Research
    on NPC: *Scientific Research*, edited by Chinese Academy
    of Medical Science (Beijing), 1975.
11. Hu Ms, et al.: *New Medicine (Canton) (12)*: 10, 1972.
12. Zeng Yi, et al.: *Journal of Chinese Oncol. 1(2)*: 81,
    1979.
13. Zeng Yi, et al.: *Journal of Chinese Oncol. 1(1)*: 2,
    1979.
14. Head and Neck Department of the Tumor Hospital of
    Chungshan Medical College: *Prevention and Treatment of
    Cancer (Canton) 2*: 23, 1972.
15. Hsieh Chih-Kuang, Li Chen-Chuan, et al.: *Chinese
    Medical Journal 84(12)*: 767, 1965.
16. Hsieh Chih-Kuang, Li chen-Chuan: Further Observation on
    Early Diagnosis and Clinical Types of Late Cases of
    Nasopharyngeal Carcinoma Based on 2,000 Cases.
    Unpublished data.
17. Fun Shun-Fa, Li Chen-Chuan: *New Medicine (Canton) (3)*:
    1980.
18. Sun Chen-Chuan, Li Chen-Chuan: Unpublished data.

Cancer Therapy

RECENT PROGRESS IN ANTINEOPLASTIC
DRUG RESEARCH IN CHINA

BIN XU
Shanghai Institute of Materia Medica
Chinese Academy of Sciences

Experimental antineoplastic drug research in China began in the mid-fifties. During the past twenty-five years several national cancer congresses have been held in Tienjin (1959, 1969), Shanghai (1962) and Beijing (1977). At these meetings the research accomplishments related to antitumor drugs were presented and summarized. In addition, some special conferences on anticancer agents were held in Shanghai (1971), Shijiazhang (1972), Beijing (1973) and Chanzher (1978)[1]. During these meetings, not only was the effectiveness of the drugs demonstrated, but also anticancer research programs were planned on a national scale. For example, in 1972 cooperative research project groups were organized to study six antitumor drugs (Camptotheca acuminata, cantharidin, Cephalotaxus, colchicine, monocrotaline and Curcuma zedoaria). In order to facilitate the research, each group was generally organized to consist of several research institutes, pharmaceutical groups and hospitals located in a number of provinces. In this paper the agents which have potential anticancer activity are summarized, and some of them are discussed briefly.

METHODOLOGICAL ASPECTS

In general the methods used for screening antitumor agents were the same as those in other countries, but some methods were modified. In the early stage Ehrlich ascites carcinoma and sarcoma 180 were very commonly employed. Later sarcoma 37, Walker carcino-sarcoma, an ascites hepatoma, Yoshida sarcoma, brain tumor-22, uterine carcinoma-14, leukemia 615 and other tumors were added. At the present time, in addition to the above tumor models, L1210, Lewis lung tumor, B16 melanoma and P388 are also used. Most recently, a cell line of a human hepatocarcinoma, SGA-73 carcinoma of the esophagus, an experimental hepatoma with positive AFP, human tumor xenografts in athymic mice and other new tumor models are being tried. The sensitivity of different tumor models and some modified screening methods have been reported elsewhere[2].

Reviewing the whole history of anticancer screening in China, it might be pointed out that there were two peaks of activity, one being around 1958 and another being about 1970. From 1958 to 1960, a large number of medicinal herbs and traditional Chinese remedies were screened in many provinces. Meanwhile, in some large cities searches for new antitumor antibiotics and new synthetic compounds were initiated. At that time about 2000 medicinal plant preparations, 300 synthetic compounds and 10,000 microbial strains (mainly streptomyces) were screened. In or about 1970 many pharmaceutical groups and hospitals began to screen anticancer agents. In the Shanghai region alone more than 1000 medicinal plants were tested. According to the data collected in the Shanghai Institute of Materia Medica, about 2000 synthetic compounds, 2000 constituents from 400 species of medicinal herbs and 460 fermentation products from microorganisms were investigated in the past 20 years. It is difficult to determine the total amount of anticancer screening which took place throughout the entire country.

Table 1. Some New Antitumor Agents in China

1. Synthetic Compounds	3. Plant Principles
Methoxysarcolysin (3P)	Camptothecin (Sodium & Suspension)
N-Formyl-sarcolysin (NF)	10-Hydroxycamptothecin
Isosarcolysin (Ho-14)	Harringtonine
Ocaphane (AT-581)	Homoharringtonine
Nitrocaphane (AT-1258)	Colchicinamide
Uraphetine	Curzerenone
Thyminalkylamine	Monocrotaline
M-25	Lycobetaine
AT-1727	Oridonin
Tisupurine (AT-1438)	Indirubin
Antimony-71 (Sb-71)	4. Miscellaneous
2. Antibiotics	Cantharidin
Actinomycin K1 and K2 (D)	Hydroxycantharidinamine
Peiyanmycin	Tilorone
Oxalysine	8 Br-cAMP

SOME NEW ANTICANCER AGENTS

A summary of potential anticancer agents is shown in Table 1. The main results concerning these compounds is presented as follows.

1. SYNTHETIC COMPOUNDS
1.1. Methoxysarcolysin (3P)[3,4]

3P or p-bis-(2-chloroethyl)-amino-o-methoxy-phenylalanine is a derivative of sarcolysin (Fig. 1). In pharmacological studies it was shown to have a strong antitumor activity on sarcoma 180, a brain tumor (B-22), Walker carcino-sarcoma and other animal tumors. It could also inhibit the leukemoid reaction in mice bearing reticulum-cell sarcoma. 3P was used orally and was easily absorbed. The highest blood concentration was attained 30 minutes after oral administration, and then the concentration dropped steadily. The drug was distributed throughout many internal organs, and the highest concentrations were found in the bone marrow, kidney and liver. About 40% of the drug was excreted in the urine during the first 24 hours, and smaller amounts were detected in feces. Methoxysarcolysin could inhibit

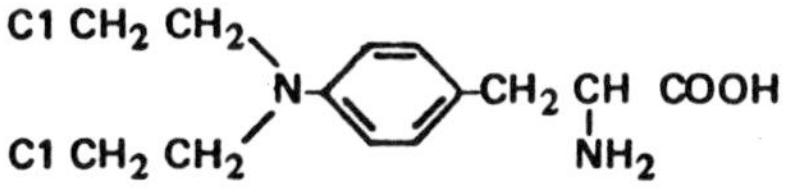

L-sarcolysin

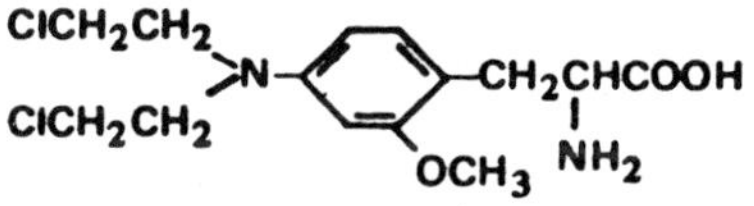

p-bis-(2-chloroethyl)-amino-0-
methoxy-phenylalanine

Methoxysarcolysin (3P)

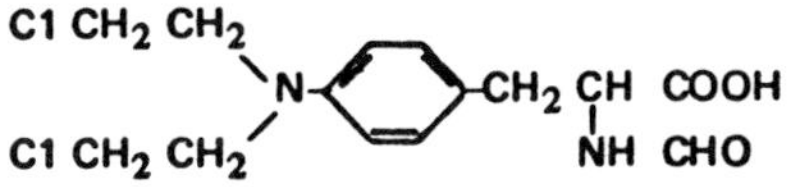

N-formyl-sarcolysin

Fig. 1 The structure of sarcolysin, methoxysarcolysin (3P) and N-formyl-sarcolysin (NF).

mitosis and nucleic acid metabolism in cancer cells. The
mechanism of its action resembled that of other alkylating
agents.

Clinical trials of this drug on 240 patients with a
variety of neoplastic diseases showed that its effectiveness
was about 41%. The best therapeutic results were obtained
in patients with chronic myelocytic leukemia. Of 40 cases,
37 were evaluated as effectively treated. In 10 cases there
was complete remission; in some of these there was no recurrence during a ten year follow-up period.

1.2. N-formyl-sarcolysin (NF) [5]

Formylsarcolysin, DL-p-bis(2-chloroethyl)amino-N-formyl-
phenylalanine has a broad antitumor spectrum, inhibiting the
growth of Yoshida sarcoma, Walker tumor, reticulum-cell
sarcoma, Krebs-2 ascites carcinoma and others. Pharmacological experiments showed that NF could inhibit protein synthe -
sis and the incorporation of ^{3}H-thymidine into nucleic acid.
Its therapeutic dose caused abnormalities in the chromosomes
of the tumor cells. By means of electron microscopy, pro-
gressive degeneration in the mitochondria and an increase in
the number of lysosomes were observed. The drug could be
administered orally, but the absorption into the gastrointestinal tract was incomplete.

Clinical observations demonstrated that NF possesses a
marked therapeutic effect on seminoma. The 5-year survival
rate was 71% when the drug was used alone. It is also used
in combination with radiation therapy or surgery.

1.3. Nitrocaphane (AT-1258) [6,7]

Nitrocaphane is chemically 2-bis-(2-chloroethyl)-amino-
methyl-5-nitro-phenylalanine. It was synthesized on the
basis of a series of studies on mechlorethamine derivatives,
including ocaphane or o-bis-(2-chloroethyl)-aminomethyl-
phenylalanine. It was hoped that the introduction of a
nitro group to the benzene ring might decrease the toxicity
of ocaphane, and thus increase its therapeutic effect (Fig.2).

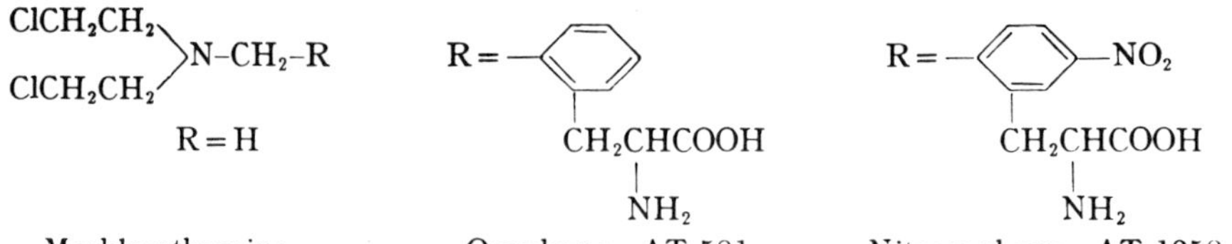

$$\begin{array}{ccc}
\text{ClCH}_2\text{CH}_2 & & \\
\qquad\qquad\qquad \text{N--CH}_2\text{--R} & R = & R = \text{---NO}_2 \\
\text{ClCH}_2\text{CH}_2 & & \\
\end{array}$$

R = H	$CH_2CHCOOH$	$CH_2CHCOOH$
	NH_2	NH_2
Mechlorethamine	Ocaphane, AT-581	Nitrocaphane, AT-1258

Fig. 2   The structures of ocaphane ((AT-581) and nitrocaphane (AT-1258)

The animal tests revealed that it has an outstanding therapeutic effect against a variety of experimental tumors. The
intraperitoneal injections of 4 mg/kg produced from 82 to 99%

inhibition of Ehrlich solid carcinoma and solid hepatoma in
mice. The therapeutic effect was nearly the same when the
drug was given orally at 8-10 mg/kg. In rats bearing 5 to 6
day-old Jensen sarcoma with 2 to 5 cm^2 of tumor mass, nitrocaphane could produce tumor regression in a majority of the
rats 12 to 15 days after seven injections of the drug, the
cure rate being from 62 to 86%.

When nitrocaphane and ocaphane were used at the same
tolerated dose, ocaphane (2 mg/kg) caused 67% and nitrocaphane (4 mg/kg) 96% (P<0.01) of tumor inhibition in mice
bearing Ehrlich carcinoma. Nitrocaphane at 1.5 mg/kg inhibited Brown-Pearce carcinoma in 66 to 78% of rabbits inoculated
intraocularly, but the inhibition caused by ocaphane was only
49 to 65%. Both compounds prolonged the survival of rabbits
(between 110 and 120%) when the tumor was inoculated intravenously. The experiments with ^{14}C-nitrocaphane demonstrated
that the radioactivity was distributed throughout many
internal organs after oral administration. The highest
content of ^{14}C was found in the kidney, lower intestine, liver,
tumor, lung and other tissues. In normal rats, the biological
halflife of the compound in plasma was about 13 minutes. It
was excreted mainly in urine and feces, 65% of the total
being excreted within 24 hours.

In clinical trials, 560 cancer patients were treated
with this drug. Among them, 443 cases were given nitrocaphane
alone; others were treated by a combination therapy with other
anticancer drugs or radiotherapy as well. The therapeutic
effect was frequently observed in carcinomas of the squamous
cell and undifferentiated cell types. This drug is more
effective against nasopharyngeal carcinoma, malignant lymphoma,
and lung cancer. It can be administered intravenously, orally
and locally. The onset of its therapeutic action was rapid,
but the duration of remission rather short, lasting about one
month. Clinical side reactions such as anorexia, vomiting,
bone marrow depression and alopecia were observed and could
be ameliorated or abolished by symptomatic treatment.

1.4. Tisurpurine (AT-1438) [8]

Tisurpurine or 6-thio-sulfonate-9 (or 7)-sodium-purine
(Fig. 3) has similar antitumor action to that of 6-mercapto-
purine. It can be easily changed into 6MP when the drug is
injected into the body, either by the action of the acid pH
of the tumor tissue or by interaction with sulfhydryl compounds. The great advantage of tisupurine is that it is
water soluble and can be injected intravenously. Clinical
trials on 170 cancer patients showed that it has remarkable
therapeutic effect against choriocarcinoma, the effective

rate being 71%. It also exerted therapeutic action on acute leukemia. For the treatment of metastatic brain malignancy, it can also be injected intrathecally.

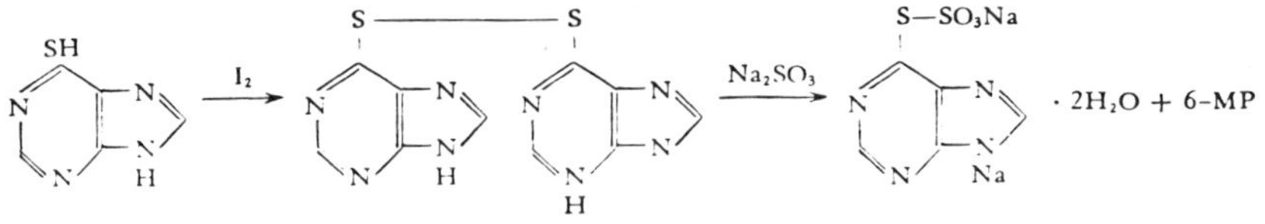

6MP   Tisupurine (AT-1438)

Fig. 3   The structures of 6-mercaptopurine (6MP) and tisupurine (AT-1438).

1.5. Antimony -71 (SB-71)[9]

In 1958-1959 Sb-71 or antimony triacetic acid (Fig. 4) was found both experimentally and clinically to be effective against some neoplasms. Based on these observations a series of studies was performed. It was demonstrated that the drug's antitumor action was mainly related to the interaction with the sulfhydryl group and zinc metabolism. At present, this drug is employed chiefly for the treatment of fibrosarcoma and gastrointestinal cancers.

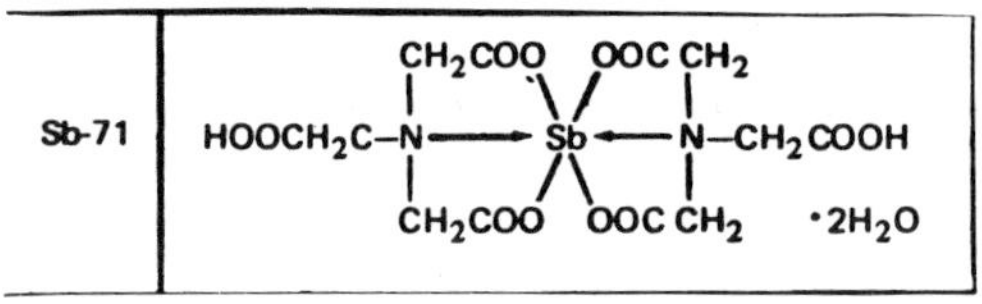

Fig. 4   The structure of
antimony ammonia
triacetic acid
(Sb-71).

1.6. Others[1,10]

Some other antitumor drugs were also investigated in China. Isosarcolysin (p-bis-(2-chloroethyl)-amino-β-phenyl-alanine) was found to be useful in treatment of malignant lymphomas, ocaphane (O-bis-(2-chloroethyl)-aminomethyl-phenylalanine) effective for treatment of the pleural effusion of lung cancer, uraphetine effective in chronic leukemia. M25 and AT-1727 were also useful anticancer agents.

2.   PLANT PRINCIPLES

2.1.   Camptothecin and hydroxycamptothecin[11-15]

Camptothecin (CPT) was tested for treatment of gastric carcinoma and other malignant diseases in the United States some years ago. Because of its side effects, it is not used now. However, in China an effort was made to decrease its toxicity and increase its effectiveness. Monoammonium glycyrrhizinate was found to be useful in decreasing the toxicity of CPT[13]. Camptothecin suspension in particle size about 1 μM was successfully made for intravenous use[16]. The drug concentration in the liver tissue was higher than that

of sodium camtothecin. Clinical trials on 450 patients
showed that camptothecin suspension had a definite therapeutic effect on liver carcinoma, increasing the percentage
of successful surgical operation from between 18% and 49%.
The one year survival rate was raised from 39% to 54%.

10-Hydroxycamptothecin (OPT) was isolated from the same
tree, Camptotheca acuminata by means of an improved method,
and a 0.002% yield from the fruits could be attained at the
Shanghai Institute of Materia Medica[17] (Fig. 5). The total
synthesis of this compound was also successfully accomplished
in China. From pharmacological experiments, OPT was found
to have a broad antitumor spectrum, inhibiting the growth of
more than 15 experimental tumors, e.g., S180, S-37, U-14,
Ehrlich carcinoma, Ascites hepatoma, Hepatoma BW 7756,
Reticulum-cell sarcoma, Walker tumor, Yoshida sarcoma, B16,
L-1210, P388, Lewis lung carcinoma, M-109 lung tumor, SC
Colon 38 and others[18-22]. It was widely distributed throughout the internal organs, and a rather high concentration was
detected in the tumor tissue. It was excreted principally
in the feces and less in the urine. Observation showed
camptothecin excretion to be quite different. OPT had
stronger inhibitory action on DNA synthesis than on RNA in
tumor cells. In the electron microscope some damage to the
tumor envelope and membrane structures were observed due to
the drug. The inhibitory action of OPT on host immunity was
not great, and it was much less when administered in a
loading dose regime, or once every four days.

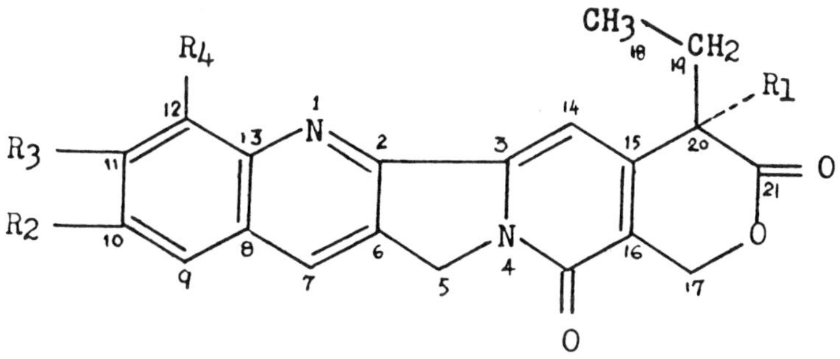

Camptothecin   R1 = OH   R2 = R3 = R4 = H

10-hydroxycamptothecin   R1 = OH   R2 = OH   R3 = R4 = H

Fig. 5   The structures of camptothecin and 10-hycroxycampto-
         thecin.

Clinical studies in 250 cancer patients revealed that
OPT was effective against primary liver carcinoma, cancer of
the head and nock, leukemia, and gastric carcinoma. The side
reactions were fewer than those caused by sodium camptothecin,
in particular the irritant action on the urinary tract was
greatly reduced.

2.2. Harringtonine and homoharringtonine[23-26]

In China harringtonine and homoharringtonine were
successfully isolated from several species of Cephalotaxus
during the past nine years (Fig. 6). Pharmacological experiments showed that cephalotaxine had no antitumor effect, but
the ester containing alkaloids, e.g., harringtonine and
homoharringtonine exhibited a definite antineoplastic
activity against animal tumors. They could inhibit protein
and nucleic acid synthesis in tumor cells. Research in cell
kinetics proved that it belongs to the class of cell cycle
nonspecific agents. After intravenous injection, the biological halflives of ^{3}H-harringtonine and ^{3}H-homoharrington-
ine in the blood were 13 and 32 minutes respectively.
Clinical data demonstrated that these two drugs could exert
a remarkable therapeutic action on acute myeloblastic
leukemia, acute monoblastic leukemia and erythroleukemia.
Tumors in some patients, which were resistant to other known
antileukemic drugs, are still sensitive to these two drugs.

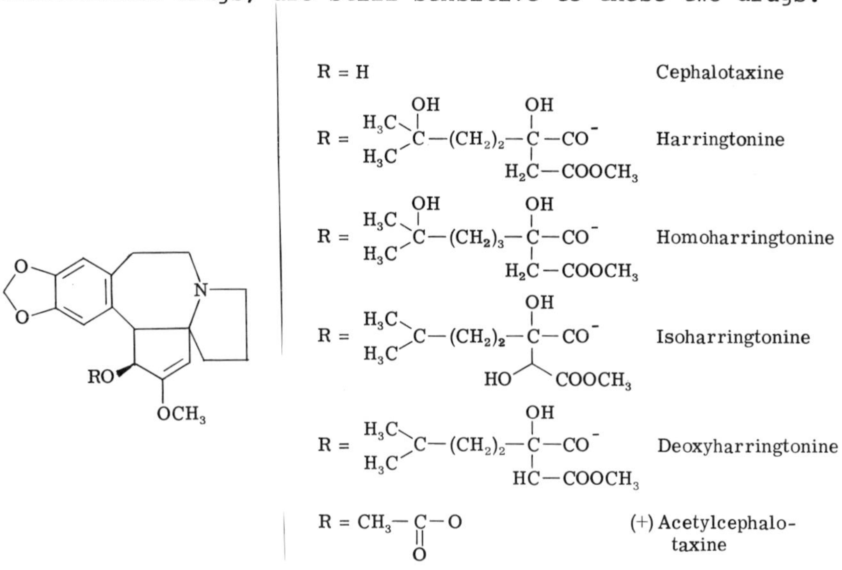

Fig. 6   The structures of harringtonine, homoharringtonine
         and other related compounds.

2.3. Colchicine and colchicinamide[1]

It is well known that colchicine has some antitumor activity. Since 1971 some institutions in the Tienjin area have been aware of this drug, and have used it in combination with other detoxifying agents. After treatment with this preparation, some patients with mammary carcinoma had a good response, and the side effects were not severe.

Colchicinamide is a derivative of colchicine prepared by using an amino group to replace the methoxy group at position 14. After pharmacological studies it was also recommended for clinical trials. Mammary carcinoma was found to be the most sensitive to the drug, its effectiveness being 74%.

2.4. Curzerenone[1]

Curzerenone is one of the main active principles isolated from Curcuma zedoaria (Berg.) Rose or Curcuma wenchowensis Sp. Nor. Pharmacological experiments revealed that it had an inhibitory effect on Ehrlich carcinoma, L615, and other tumors. Clinical trials showed that it is effective against carcinoma of the uterine cervix and skin carcinoma.

2.5. Monocrotaline[1]

In Chinese folk medicine Crotalaria sessiflora was used to treat skin and cervical carcinomas. From chemical and pharmacological studies monocrotaline was found to be the active principle. It inhibited the growth of experimental animal tumors, but in human patients, due to its hepatic toxicity, its use was limited.

2.6. Lycobetaine[27]

In Chinese traditional medical literature Lycoris radiata Herb. was described to have some actions resembling tumor-inhibiting effects, but experimental screening of its major components could not demonstrate any effective antitumor substance. When its main alkaloid lycorine was changed into lycobetaine, the antineoplastic action could be demonstrated. Lycobetaine was shown to possess a noticeable antitumor action on several animal tumors such as Ehrlich carcinoma, ascites hepatoma, sarcoma 180 and Yoshida sarcoma. It was also effective when injected intragastrically. The study of structure-activity relationships showed that the antitumor action was closely related to its betaine structure (Fig. 7).

Lycobetaine has been tried on 230 cancer patients and was shown to be effective in gastric carcinoma and ovarian carcinoma.

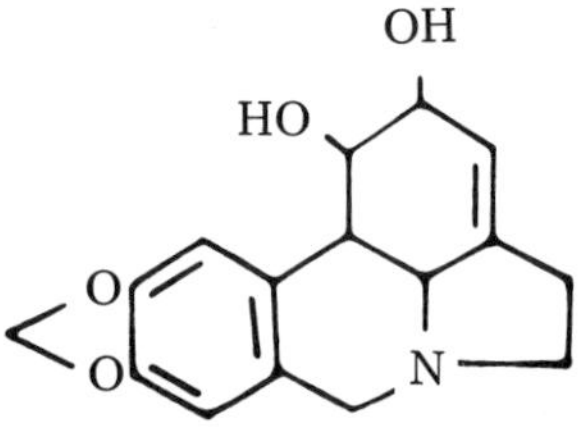

Lycorine 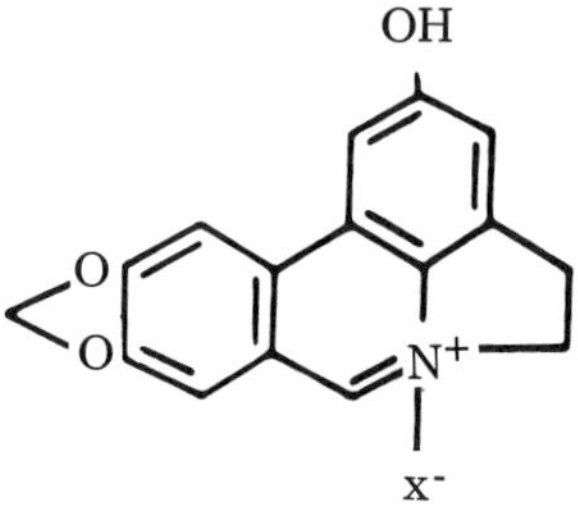   AT-1840   x = CH_3COO or Cl

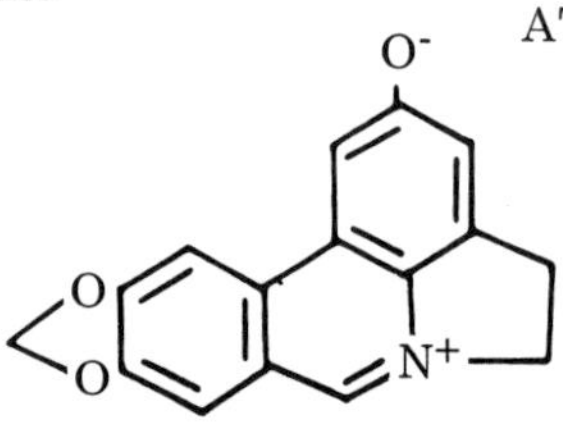

Free base lycobetaine

Fig. 7 The structures of lycorine and lycobetaine.

2.7. Oridonin[28]

In folk medicine, Rabdosia rubeseus Hamst was used in some provinces of China to treat carcinomas of the esophagus and stomach. It contains a variety of terpenes. After screening, oridonin was demonstrated to be the main active principle. In mice it exhibited an inhibitory action on sarcoma 180 and on ascites hepatoma. Clinical trials revealed that this agent could exert a palliative action on the symptoms of esophageal cancer and cardiac and stomach carcinomas. A therapeutic effect on severe hyperplasia of esophageal epithelia was observed as well.

2.8. Indirubin[1]

Two famous plants, Baphicacanthes cusia Bremek and Indigofera tinctoria L., have been employed in Chinese traditional medical practices for a long time. Remission was observed in some leukemia patients receiving such plant preparations. In experimental animals some components of this preparation were effective in Walker tumor syndrome. After systematic analysis, indirubin was proved to be the main principle possessing therapeutic effect on chronic

myelocytic leukemia. The synthetic compound has the same
effect as the natural one. In some instances nausea, diar-
rhea and other side effects were noticed.

Apart from the above mentioned compounds, some other
plants and ingredients, such as Grifola umbellata, Poria
cocos, Stephania tetrandra S. Moore, Allium sativum L.,
Acanthopanax senticosus Harm., Pinellia pedatisecta Schott
and Maytanus were also found to have some antineoplastic
activity. Much work, however, is still to be done.

3. ANTIBIOTICS

Between 1956 and 1957, the antitumor antibiotic actinomycin K was discovered in China [29-32]. After a series of
investigations, it was found that actinomycin K consisted of
two components. K-2 is identical with actinomycin D, while
K-1 is a new actinomycin containing glycine in its peptide
chain of the structure. The former is manufactured with the
name kensenmycin, and is used in the treatment of a variety
of neoplastic diseases, particularly for choriocarcinoma and
chorioadenoma. K-1 was found to be less active, so it was
not recommended for clinical trial. Some well known antibiotics, such as mitomycin, mithramycin, rubidomycin, bleomycin and streptonigrin were also investigated during the
past 20 years. Micro organisms producing these antibiotics
were discovered in Chinese soil some years ago. After
completion of chemical and pharmacological studies, there
was some production of these antibiotics. At the present
time two antibiotics, i.e. peiyanmycin and oxalysine, are
still under investigation.

3.1. Peiyanmycin[1]

Peiyanmycin belongs to the class of glyco-peptide antibiotics isolated from the soil in Peiyan county of the
Chiejian province. It can inhibit SGA-73 carcinoma of the
esophagus in mice, and its pulmonary toxicity was found to
be less than that of bleomycin A-2. Clinical data showed it
to have a therapeutic effect on carcinoma of the head and
neck, being 70% effective. It is also effective in nasopharyngeal, mammary and esophageal carcinomas.

3.2. Oxalysine (I-677)[33-35]

L-4-oxalysine (Fig. 8), a new antibiotic, was isolated
from Streptomyces roseoviridofuscus n. sp., and found to have
a remarkable inhibitory action on the solid forms of several
animal tumors, but no significant influence on ascites forms.
When it was used in combination with lysine, the antitumor

action disappeared or diminished. I-677 diminished markedly
the blood fibrinogen level, which might be related to the
tumor metastasis. Therefore, the mechanism of its antitumor
action might be different from other anticancer drugs.

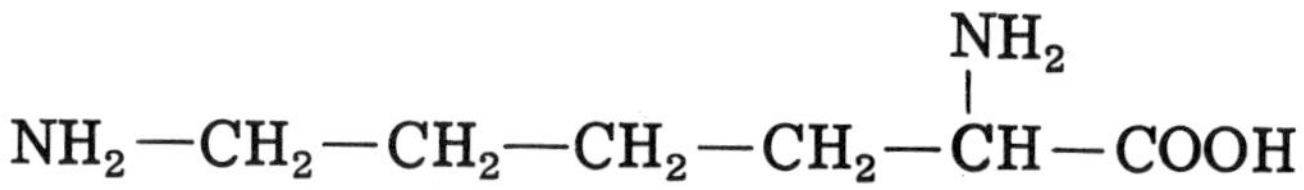

$$NH_2-CH_2-CH_2-CH_2-CH_2-\overset{\overset{\displaystyle NH_2}{|}}{CH}-COOH$$

Lysine

$$NH_2-CH_2-CH_2-O-CH_2-\overset{\overset{\displaystyle NH_2}{|}}{CH}-COOH$$

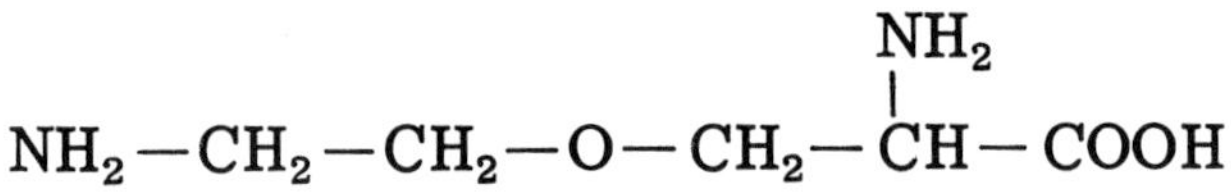

L-4-oxalysine

Fig. 8 The structures of lysine and L-4-oxalysine.

Clinically the drug has been tested on about 30 cancer
patients. Preliminary results showed that oxalysine had
certain beneficial effects on metastatic liver carcinoma,
improving the liver function of patients with high GPT level,
and relieving other symptoms as well. It was also used for
the treatment of patients with chronic persistent hepatitis.
The GPT level of about 70% of the patients returned to normal
after the drug was administered.

4. *MISCELLANEOUS*[1]

In China some new types of anticancer agents have
attracted the attention of oncologists. For instance, the
antitumor action of tilorone, poly(I).poly(C), interferon-
inducers, bromo-cAMP, poly-saccharides from Bacterium
Prodigiosum and mushrooms were investigated. Some of them
are now at the stage of clinical trials.
Cantharidin, a known chemical compound (Fig. 9), was
isolated from Mylabris phalerata pall., a kind of bettle[36].
Because the beetle was employed for the treatment of

malignant diseases for a long time in folk medicine, this highly active substance, cantharidin, has been studied extensively in China in recent years. Animal experiments showed cantharidin to possess a definite antineoplastic effect on several experimental tumors. It was easily adsorbed by injection or oral administration. The drug concentration was rather high in the intestine, stomach, liver, and tumor tissue. Its therapeutic dose exhibited no obvious suppressive effect on host immunity. In clinical study cantharidin was used in an oral dose of between 0.25 and 2 mg daily for 1 to 2 months without marked side reactions. The therapeutic effects were observed in patients with primary hepatocarcinoma, intestinal carcinoma and other neoplasms.

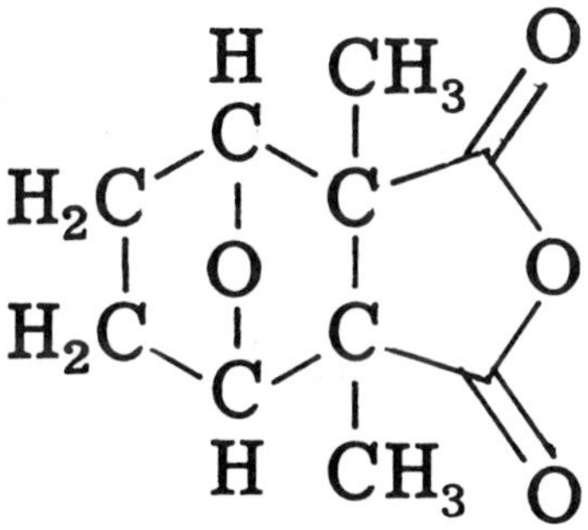

Fig. 9   The structure of cantharidin.

Some derivatives of cantharidin, e.g., hydroxycanthari-dinamine, methylcantharidin, and sodium cantharidin, were investigated recently. They were also found to have anti-tumor activity.

SUMMARY

From the above twenty or more antineoplastic agents, it can be seen that the chemists and pharmacologists, in cooperation with other experts, have made some progress in anticancer drug research. In this paper, a brief account of these accomplishments is given. The details of the chemistry, pharmacology and clinical studies concerning these drugs are reported elsewhere. At the present time, the mortality rates of cancer in some areas of China are among the highest and the problem of a search for new, highly effective anticancer drugs is still a very important task. Undoubtedly, more efforts to study Chinese traditional medicinal drugs and to develop new leads will help in the discovery of such drugs.

REFERENCES

1. Xu (Hsu), B. and Han, J.: Recent developments in the studies of anticancer drugs. *Chinese J. Oncology (Zhonghua Zhongliu Zazhi) 1:* 315, 1979.
2. Hsu, B. et al.: Studies on the sensitivity of several tumor models in screen of anticancer agents. *Kexue Tongbao (Scientia) 20:* 242, 1975.
3. Chen, J.T., Hsu, B., et al.: Studies on antitumor drugs. Vl. Experimental therapy and toxicity of p-bis(2-chloro-ethyl)amino-o-methoxy-phenylalanine (3P). *Acta Pharm. Sinica 8:* 217, 1960.
4. Hsu, B., Kao, Y.S., et al.: Pharmacological studies of several new antitumor agents. *Scientia Sinica 13:* 789, 1964. (English ed.)
5. Han, J., Wang, C.K., et al.: Effect of N-formyl-sarco-lysin on experimental tumors. *Chinese Med. J. 81:* 574, 1962. (English ed.)
6. Shanghai Institute of Materia Medica, et al.: Antitumor studies on nitrocaphane (AT-1258). *Chinese Med. J. 54:* 693, 1974.
7. Chou, C.H., Hsu, B., et al.: The absorption, distribution and excretion of nitrocaphane (AT-1258). *Chinese Med. J. 57:* 158, 1977.
8. Shanghai Institute of Materia Medica, et al.: The anti-tumor action of tisupurine (AT-1438). *Scientia Sinica (2),* 281, 1977.
9. Hsu, B., Chou, C.H., et al.: Studies on antitumor action of antimony-complexones. *Acta Un. Int. Cancer 20:* 245, 1964.
10. Li, C.P.: Anticancer agents recently developed in the People's Republic of China. *DHEW Publication,* Washington, D.C. 1974.
11. Wall, M.E., et al.: Plant antitumor agent 1. The isolation and structure of Camptothecin, a novel alkaloidal leukemia and tumor inhibitor from Camptotheca acuminata. *J. Am. Chem. Soc. 88:* 3888, 1966.
12. Wani, M.C., et al.: Plant antitumor agents II. The structure of two new alkaloids from Camptotheca acuminata. *J. Org. Chem. 34:* 364, 1969.
13. Shanghai Institute of Materia Medica, Department of Pharmacology: Experimental study of the anticancer action of camptothecin. *Chinese Med. J. 55:* 274, 1975.
14. Lin, L.T., et al.: Chemical constituents of the anti-cancer plant Camptotheca acuminata Decne 1. Chemical constituents of the roots of Camptotheca acuminata Decne. *Acta Chimica Sinica 35:* 227, 1977.

15. Moertel, C.G., et al.: Phase II study of camptothecin (NSC-100880) in the treatment of advanced gastrointestinal cancer. *Cancer Chemother. Rep. 56:* 95, 1972.

16. Shanghai Institute of Materia Medica et al.: Studies on intravenous injection of camptothecin suspensoid in treatment of liver carcinoma and leukemia. *Kexue Tongbao 22:* 552, 1977.

17. Hsu, J.S., et al.: Chemical constituents of the anti-cancer plant Camptotheca acuminata Decne II. Chemical constituents of the fruits of Camptotheca acuminata Decne. *Acta Chimica Sinica 35:* 193, 1977.

18. Shanghai Institute of Materia Medica, Academia Sinica: Studies on the anticancer action of 10-hydroxycamptothecin. *Chinese Med. J. (10):* 598, 1978.

19. Wang, T.W., Hsu, B., et al.: The influence of 10-hydroxycamptothecin on the ultrastructure of ascites hepatoma cells in mice. *Chinese J. Oncology 1:* 183, 1979.

20. Hsu, B., Miller, E.E., Lo, K.W., and Tsou, K.C.: Anti-tumor effect of 10-hydroxycamptothecin on mouse hepatoma BW 7756 and its possible mechanism of action. To be published, 1980.

21. The U.S. National Cancer Institute: Data report on the antitumor activity of 10-hydroxycamptothecin. Personal communication, 1979.

22. Gordon, M.: Data report of Bristol Laboratories on the anticancer tests of 10-hydroxycamptothecin (NSC 107024) and other compounds. Personal communication, 1979,1980.

23. Powell, R.G., et al.: Antitumor alkaloids from Cephalotaxus harringtonia structure and activity. *J. Pharm. Sci. 61:* 1227, 1972.

24. Ma, G.E., et al.: Studies on the alkaloids of Cephalotaxus fortunei. *Acta Chimica Sinica 35:* 201, 1977.

25. Xu, B., Chen, J.T., et al.: New results in pharmacologic research of some anticancer agents. U.S.-China Pharmacology Symposium, Washington, D.C. October 29-31, 1979.

26. Ji, X.J., et al.: Mechanism of action of harringtonine, a new anticancer agent. ibid, 1979.

27. Owen, T.Y., et al. A new antitumor substance -- lyco-betaine (AT-1840). *Kexue Tongbao 21:* 285, 1976.

28. Honan Institute of Medical Science, Department of Pharmaceutical Chemistry, et al.: A new antitumor substance -- rubescensine. *Kexue Tongbao 23:* 53, 1978.

29. Tsai, J.S., Hsu, B., et al.: Actinomycin K -- a new antitumor substance. *Scientia (23):* 717, 1957.

30. Hsu, B., et al.: Actinomycin K -- an antibiotic
    against tumor. *Chinese Med. J. 78:* 413, 1959 (English
    ed.)
31. Department of Obstetrics and Gynecology, Peking Fanti
    Hospital: Treatment of choriocarcinoma and chorioadenoma
    destruens by chemotherapy and surgery: 226 consecutive
    cases in 7 years. *China's Med. (4):* 294, 1967 (English
    ed.)
32. Hsu, B., et al.: Studies on the mechanism of antitumor
    action of actinomycin K. *Scientia Sinica 12:* 535,1963.
33. Yueh, H.F., et al.: The antitumor action of oxalysine
    (I-677), a new antibiotic. *Kexue Tongbao 24:* 47, 1979.
34. Zhang, H.L., Wu, S.Y., et al.: Studies on the anti-
    metabolic antibiotics I. Taxonomic study on L-4-oxalysine
    producer -- Streptomyces roseoviridofuscus n. sp.
    Acta Microbiologica Sinica 19: 126, 1979.
35. Li, H.Y., et al.: Pharmacological studies of oxalysine
    on experimental hepatitis. *Acta Biochimica et Biophysica
    Sinica 11:* 151, 1979.
36. Chen, J.T., et al.: Studies on the pharmacological
    actions of cantharidin. *Chinese Med. J. 57:* 475, 1977.

GENE AMPLIFICATION IN METHOTREXATE RESISTANT CELLS[+]

J.R. BERTINO,[*] B. DOLNICK, R. BERENSON,[**]
B.A. KAMEN,[***] D.I. SCHEER

*Departments of Medicine and Pharmacology,
Yale University School of Medicine
and the Department of Biology,
Yale University, New Haven, Conn.*

Development of many effective anticancer agents in the past two decades has resulted in a marked improvement in drug treatment of cancer. It is now possible to achieve temporary remissions in several cancers, and even cure in a few using chemotherapeutic agents. Despite the use of drug combinations, most cancers eventually become refractory to chemotherapy, and the development of drug resistance within tumor preparations remains a major obstacle to successful drug treatment of malignancy.[1,2]

A wide variety of biochemical mechanisms have been demonstrated, whereby tumor cells become resistant to anticancer drugs.[3] Methotrexate (MTX), an important and widely used chemotherapeutic agent, has been especially well studied from this view point, and both cytogenetic as well as biochemical changes have been described for highly resistant tumor cell lines, propagated *in vitro*.

Three different mechanisms associated with development of drug resistance in experimental systems, have been described: impairment of transport of MTX; an increase in the target enzyme for MTX, dihydrofolate reductase (DHFR); or an altered DHFR, with decreased affinity for MTX (reviewed in 4). Cell lines have also been described that have two alterations; e.g., an elevated DHFR and impaired MTX transport.[6]

Because these mammalian cell lines may be made highly resistant to MTX, these alterations may be exaggerated and therefore studies of the molecular mechanisms responsible for these events become easier to identify and characterize.

---

*American Cancer Society Professor
**Current Address: Dept. of Medicine, University of Utah
School of Medicine, Salt Lake City, Utah
***Current Address: Children's Hospital, Milwaukee, WI
+Supported by Grants CA08010 from the USPHS

IMPAIRED MTX TRANSPORT

Several mammalian lines have now been described that transport MTX poorly, or not at all.[6-10] One such line, carefully studied,[11] was found to virtually exclude MTX; the small amount of radiolabel that did enter the cell was shown to be almost entirely composed of MTX breakdown products. We have postulated that impaired MTX transport does not occur *in vivo*, since cells must be able to transport reduced folates (the natural substances that interact with the membrane carrier) for survival.[12] *In vitro*, such cells can survive, since most tissue culture media contains high concentrations of folic acid, which enters cells by a different transport system than does reduced folates.[13] Thus far, the nature of this transport defect has not been elucidated. It is of interest that resistance to vincalkaloids has been found to be associated with changes in membrane glycoprotein concentrations and, in one cell line, a cytogenetic change as well (increase in a homogenous staining region on a marker chromosome).[14] How these changes relate to the altered MTX transport system is under extensive study.

ALTERATION OF BINDING AFFINITY FOR MTX BY DHFR

A few examples have been described of tumor cell lines resistant to MTX by virtue of an alteration in DHFR resulting in decreased binding to MTX.[5,15,16] Flintoff, et al.[5] have developed lines with both an elevated DHFR and an altered DHFR enzyme, that are highly resistant to MTX.[5,16] The nature of the presumed change(s) in the amino acid content of the enzyme and in the corresponding nucleotide sequence in the gene resulting in this enzyme alteration has not been elucidated as yet.

ELEVATED LEVELS OF DHFR

When cells are exposed to low concentrations of MTX, and the surviving cells are exposed to increased concentrations of this drug in stepwise fashion, highly resistant cell lines may be obtained (e.g. 100,000 fold). When these cells are examined for associated biochemical changes, an elevated level of DHFR activity is commonly observed.[17-23] Thus, we and others have obtained MTX resistant lines with 200-1000 fold elevations of this enzyme (Table 1).

The question of how cells are able to synthesize high levels of DHFR has been resolved recently.[20,22,26] When cell lines have been examined that have an increased level of DHFR,

TABLE I

Relative Levels of DHFR, mRNA, and Gene Dosage in MTX Resistant Cell Lines

Cell Lines	Relative DHFR* Activity	Rate of DHFR** Synthesis	Relative DHFR* mRNA	Relative DHFR** Gene Dosage	Reference
(1) Sarcoma 180 A-3000	250	5.9 %	220	180	(22,23)
(2) L1210 L1210 RR	35	2.2 %	35	45	(22,23)
(3) L5178Y L5178R	300	10.12 %	300	300	(20)
(4) CHO MK42	240	4.1 %	---	150	(24)
(5) 3T6 - R_1	---	3.3 %	30	35	(25)
3T6 - R_2	---	10.4 %	> 90	100	

*Relative to parent sensitive line

**% DHFR in sensitive or parent line less than 0.1%

all of them have been found to have a corresponding increase in the rate of synthesis of this enzyme, with a corresponding increase in the amount of mRNA coding for DHFR (Table 1).

Surprisingly, this increase in DHFR activity is presumably a consequence of an increased number of (amplified) genes coding for this enzyme activity.[22] Several mammalian lines have now been shown to have increases in gene copies of DHFR proportionate to an increase in enzyme activity (Table 1). Both stable and unstable lines with amplified DHFR genes occur. The unstable lines gradually lose DHFR activity and gene copies when propagated in the absence of the drug.[27,28]

In some instances, unstable lines were found to contain double minute (DM) chromosomes, and the level of DHFR was correlated with the number of DM chromosomes, in the cells. Based on these observations Kaufman et al.[28] suggested that some unstable lines contained DHFR genes in DM chromosomes; these were lost rapidly during cultivation in MTX-free media. In other circumstances, resistance to MTX and amplified DHFR genes were found to be associated with the appearance of a specific chromosome abnormality. These resistant cells contained a homogeneous staining region (HSR) when stained by the trypsin-giemsa method.[20,23,29] Although this change was usually associated with stable resistance, some lines were unstable and this region decreased in size as the cells lost MTX resistance.[29]

In situ hybridization studies, utilizing a [3]H cDNA probe prepared from DHFR mRNA from an MTX-resistant S-180 line, have shown that the chromosome containing the HSR in both resistant CHO line and a L5178Y line (the No. 2 chromosome in both situations) contains most or all of the amplified DHFR genes.[20,24] The size of the HSR is estimated to contain 3-5% of the total DNA in both all lines, equivalent to 2.3×10^8 base pairs. Thus, if the number of gene copies is approximately 300 as in the L5178Y line,[20] then each repeat unit is approximately 800 kbp in size. Recent evidence indicates that the DHFR gene is at least 42 kbp in size.[30,31] Thus, a great deal of additional information is represented in the other sequences in the amplified unit.[30,32] Furthermore, the DHFR gene has a minimum of 5 intervening sequences as revealed by restriction enzyme analysis. In one cell line, resistant to MTX and characterized by a 1000 fold increase in the enzyme DHFR, the HSR was shown to contain a substantial amount (60%) of highly repetitive sequences.[31]

GENE AMPLIFICATION AND DRUG RESISTANCE

Resistance of bacteria to chloramphenicol and penicillin occurs via an amplification of genes present in episomal elements, e.g., plasmids that confer the characteristic phenotype.[33,34] Although amplification of DHFR genes causing MTX resistance was the first demonstration that this mechanism could occur in mammalian cells, several other instances of elevated enzyme activity associated with resistance to various drugs are known (Table 11) and in one of these circumstances, resistance to PALA, the aspartate transcarbamylase inhibitor, has been shown to be due to amplification of the gene coding for this enzyme activity.[35,36] Thus, it appears that gene amplification is not unique to MTX resistance, and may turn out to be an important component of drug resistance generally.

In patients whose tumors become resistant to MTX, relatively little is known of cellular mechanisms. Two patients with acute lymphatic leukemia (ALL) with apparent altered affinity for MTX have been described that were clinically resistant to this drug.[1] One patient with ALL, also resistant to MTX was reported to have increased levels of DHFR.[41] Since increased levels of DHFR result from apparent stabilization of this enzyme and protection from degradation in human blood cells,[42] it is difficult to separate this phenomenon from an increase in enzyme synthesis due to gene amplification; thus, verification of amplified DHFR causing resistance in human situation will require sensitive methods (e.g. nucleic acid hybridization) that unequivocally show an increase in gene copies for DHFR. Clearly, amplification will not be of the magnitude noted in the cells cultivated *in vitro*.

CONCLUSIONS

Studies of the ways in which cells become resistant to folate antagonists have led to important insights into fundamental cellular processes. Of most interest is the notion that under selective pressure of MTX, cells may respond by amplifying the gene copies coding for the target enzyme DHFR. How this event occurs and how a cell can revert to a state of decreased number of gene copies are important questions that are being addressed with modern molecular biological techniques. The large number of gene copies as well as mRNA and enzyme synthesized, also provide a system for studying gene regulation and transcription in cells. An exciting

TABLE II

Examples of Increased Enzyme Activity Associated With Drug Resistance

Drug	Elevated Enzyme	Gene Amplification	Reference
MTX	Dihydrofolate Reductase	Yes	(20,22)
PALA	Asparate Transcarbamylase	Yes	(36)
Hydroxyurea	Ribonucleotide Reductase	N.D.*	(37)
Pyrazafurin	Orotidylic Decarboxylase	N.D.	(38)
Methylornithine	Ornithine Decarboxylase	N.D.	(39)
5-fluorodeoxyuridine	Thymidylate Synthetase	N.D.	(40)

*Not determined

derivative of this research has been the use of DNA containing amplified genes together with methotrexate selection to "transform" other donor cells to a state of MTX resistance[32,43,44] This approach offers promise for creating drug resistance in normal marrow stem cells; thus allowing more MTX to be administered to patients with malignancy, as well as a method for introducing additional genes (i.e., co-transformation) into recipient cells.[45,46]

REFERENCES

1. Skeel, R.T. and Bertino, J.R. *Proc. 5th Int. Congr. Pharmacology,* San Francisco (1972).
2. Skipper, H.E., Shabel, F.M. and Lloyd, H.H. Semin *Hematol. 15:* 207-219 (1978).
3. Brochman, R.W. In: A.C. Sartorelli and D.G. Johns (eds), Handbook of Experimental Pharmacology. Bellin and Springer (1977).
4. Bertino, J.R. *Cancer Research 39:* 293-304 (1979).
5. Flintoff, W.F., Davidson, S.V. and Siminovitch, L. Som *Cell Genet. 2:* 245-261 (1976).
6. Lindquist, C. Ph.D. Thesis, Yale University School of Medicine (1979).
7. Fisher, G.A. *Biochem. Pharmacol. 11:* 1233-1234 (1960).
8. Hakala, M.T. *Biochem. Biophys. Acta 102:* 198-209 (1965).
9. Sirotnak, F.M., Kurita, S. and Hutchison, D.J. *Cancer Research, 28:* 75-80 (1968).
10. Jackson, R.C., Niethammer, D. and Huennekens, F.M. *Cancer Biochem. Biophys.1:* 154-155 (1975).
11. Kamen, B.A., Cashmore, A.R., Dreyer, R.N., Moroson, B.A., Hsieh, P. and Bertino, J.R. *J. Biol. Chem. 255:* 3254-3257(1980).
12. Bertino, J.R., Dolnick, B.J., Berenson, R.J., Scheer, D.E. and Kamen, B.A. *Proc. 2nd Bristol Symposium,* in press.
13. Huennekens, F.M., Vitols, K.S. and Henderson, G.B. Adv. Enzymol.
14. Biedler, J.L., and Peterson, R.H.F. Bristol Symposium.
15. Albrecht, A.M., Biedler, J.L. and Hutchison, D.,. *Cancer Research 32:* 1539-1546 (1972).
16. Gupta, R.S., Flintoff, W.F. and Siminovitch, L. *Can. J. Biochem. 55:* 445-452 (1977).
17. Fisher, G.A. *Biochem. Pharmacol. 7:* 75-80 (1961).
18. Hakala, M.T., Zakrewski, S.F. and Nichol, C.A. *J. Biol. Chem. 236:* 952-958 (1961).
19. Biedler, J.L., Albrecht, A.M., Spanger, B.A. *Genetics 77:* 4-5-(1974).
20. Dolnick, B.J., Berenson, R.J., Bertino, J.R., Kaufman, R.J., Nunberg, J.H., Schimke, R.T. *J. Cell Biol. 83:* 394-402 (1979).
21. Bostock, C.J., Clark, E.M., Harding, N.G.L., Mounts, P.M., Tyler-Smith, C., Heyningen, M. and Walker, P.M.P. *Chromosoma 74:* 153-177(1979).
22. Alt, F.W., Kellems, R.E., Bertino, J.R. and Schimke, R.T. *J. Biol. Chem. 253:* 1357-1370 (1978).

23. Alt, F.W., Kellems, R.E. and Schimke, R.T. *J. Biol. Chem. 251:* 3063-3074 (1976).

24. Nunberg, J.H., Kaufman, R.J., Schimke, R.T., Urlaub, G.and Chasin, L.A. *Proc. Nat. Acad. Sci.USA 75:* 5553 (1978).

25. Kellems, R.E., Morhenn, V.B., Pfendt, E.A., Celt, F.W. and Schimke, R.T. *J. Biol. Chem. 254:* 309(1979).

26. Schimke, R.T., Alt, F.W., Kellems, R.E., Kaufman, R.J. and Bertino, J.R. *Quant. Biol. 42:* 649-658 (1977).

27. Kaufman, R.J., Bertino, J.R. and Schimke, R.T. *J. Biol. Chem. 253:* 5852-5860 (1978).

28. Kaufman, R.J., Bertino, J.R. and Schimke, R.T. *Proc. Nat. Acad. Sci. USA 76:* 5667-5673 (1979).

29. Biedler, J.L., and Splenger, B.A. *Science 191:* 185-187 (1976).

30. Nunberg, J.H., Kaufman, R.J., Chang, A.C.Y., Cohen, S.N. and Schimke, R.T. *Cell 19:* 355-364 (1980).

31. Bostock, C.J. and Clark, E.M. *Cell 19:* 709-715 (1980).

32. Scheer, D.I., Srimatkandada, S., Kamen, B.A. and Bertino J.R. Trends in Human Leukemia (1980), in press.

33. Perlman, D. and Rowand, R.H. *J. Bact. 123:* 1013 (1975).

34. Normark, S., Edlund, T., Grundstom, T., Bergstrom, S. and Wolfwatz, S. *J. Bact. 132:* 912 (1977).

35. Kempe, T.D., Swyryd, E.A., Bruist, M. and Stark, G.R. *Cell 9:* 541-550 (1976).

36. Wahl, G.M., Padgett, R.A. and Stark, G.R. *J. Biol. Chem. 254:* 8679-8689 (1979).

37. Lewis, W.H., Kuzin, B.A. and Wright, J.N. *Cell Physiol. 94:* 287 (1978).

38. Suttle, D.P. and Stark, G.R. *J. Biol. Chem. 254:* 4602 (1979).

39. Namont, P.S., Duchesne, M.C., Grove, J. and Tardif, C. *Exp. Cell Res. 115:* 387 (1978).

40. Priest, D.G. and Ledford, B.E. *Biochem. Pharmacol. 29:* 1549-1553 (1980).

41. Hryniuk, W.M. and Bertino, J.R. *J. Clin. Invest. 48:* 2140-2155 (1969).

42. Bertino, J.R. *Cancer Research 23:* 1286-1306 (1963).

43. Wigler, M., Perucho, M., Kurtz, D., Dana, S., Pellicer, A., Axel, R. and Silverstein, S. *Proc. Natl. Acad. Sci. USA 77:* 3567-3570 (1980).

44. Lewis, W.H., Srinivasan, P.R., Stokoe, N. and Siminovitch, L. *Somatic Cell Genetics 6:* 333-348 (1980).

45. Cline, M.J., Stang, H., Mercola, K. Morse, L., Rubrecht, R., Browne, J. and Salser, W. *Nature, London 284:* 422 (1980).

46. Merola, K.E., Stang, H.D., Browne, J., Salser, W. and Cline, M.J. *Science 208:* 1033-1035 (1980).

STUDIES ON HARRINGTONINE AS A NEW ANTITUMOR DRUG

PAN ZHENKUN, CHANG ZHONGYI, WANG YONGCHAO,
LEE KUN, SZE CHIANGYI, JI XIUJUAN, XU YUTING,
LI ZHANRONG AND HAN JUI
*Institute of Materia Medica, Chinese Academy
of Medical Sciences, Beijing, China*

Recently, Powell and his colleagues reported that they had isolated several alkaloids from Cephalotaxus harringtonia, and that some of these alkaloids showed significant activity in rodent tumors. However, no further pharmacological and clinical reports have been found in available literature. The beneficial effects of Cephalotaxus fortunei Hook F in the treatment of malignant growths have also been described by folk medical practitioners in Fujian Province, China. By referring to the chemotaxonomic principles and the experiences of folk medicine, we have been engaged in the botanical, chemical, pharmacological and clinical studies of Cephalotaxus hainanensis Li, which belongs to the same genus, but is of a different species from C. harringtonia.

The biological activity and clinical effectiveness of harringtonine, which is an active principle of the alkaloids isolated from the plant, will be described.

A. PHARMACOLOGICAL STUDIES

1. *ACTION ON THE TRANSPLANTABLE TUMORS:*

The methods for tumor inoculation and drug administration, and the criteria for evaluating tumor inhibition, were the same as those described previously. Experiments demonstrated that Cephalotaxine per se was inactive, while the four esters of Cephalotaxine (harringtonine, homoharringtonine, isoharringtonine and deoxyharringtonine) were active in rodent tumors. It is interesting that hainanolide (a lactone) exhibited definite activity in rodent tumors.

2. *TOXICOLOGICAL STUDIES:*

By means of conventional preclinical toxicological methods, the acute toxicity of harringtonine and three allied esters of Cephalotaxine was determined on mice. The subacute toxicity of harringtonine was studied on dogs. Experiments revealed that the LD_{50} of these four esters of Cephalotaxine varied mardedly.

    Subacute toxicological studies showed that for harring-
tonine, the maximum tolerated dosage for dogs was 0.2 mg/kg.
With a dosage in this range, the blood picture was lowered
moderately with no noticeable effects on the gastrointestinal
system, liver or renal function and ECG. With a smaller dosage, (0.1 mg/kg), harringtonine caused a slight leukopenia
and moderate thrombocytopenia in dogs. No other side-effects
were observed.

3. *EFFECT OF HARRINGTONINE ON THE MORPHOLOGY AND MITOTIC
INDEX OF L-1210 CELLS:*
    (1) Conventional Microscopical Studies
    L-1210 cells were smeared and stained by the usual meth-
od. Experiments showed that at therapeutic dosage, there
was a significant lowering of the mitotic index of the tumor
cells. Karyopyknosis, or karyorrhexis, was observed on some
of the tumor cells
    (2) Fluorescence Microscopy
    The L-1210 cells were stained with 0.02% Acridin orange
and examined by fluorescence microscope. The tumor cells of
the treated group showed a similar change to when they were
examined in conventional microscopical studies, i.e., karyopyknosis or karyorhexis.

4. *EFFECT OF HARRINGTONINE ON THE ULTRASTRUCTURE OF L-1210
CELLS:*
    The conventional methods of fixation, dehydration,
staining and ultrasection were used. Electron microscopical
studies showed that the L-1210 cells were rich in microvilli,
with large irregular nuclei and 1 to 2 nucleoli.
    There were abundant spherical or oval mitochondria in
the cytoplasm. The density varied significantly in these
mitochondria. The endoplasmic reticulum was mainly smooth-
surfaced. The cytoplasm was rich in free ribosomes. The
Golgi apparatus was well developed. As well, many virus
particles were found in the cytoplasm, and the mitotic
figures were easily encountered.
    Five hours after a single intraperitoneal injection of
harringtonine at a dosage of 1 mg/kg, the most significant
morphological change was observed in the nuclei of leukemic
cells. Initially, the chromatin was condensed in the area
near the nuclear membrane. Then, this condensed chromatin
bulged into the cytoplasm with the nuclear membrane; and
finally, the nuclear membrane was broken and resulted in
karyorrhexis (so-called apoptosis). The numbers of ribosomes
and virus particles in the cytoplasm were reduced

significantly. The smooth-surfaced endoplasmic reticula
were dilated, and lysosomes appeared. Some of these treated
leukemic cells showed cytolysis.

5. *EFFECT OF HARRINGTONINE ON THE BIOSYNTHESIS OF PROTEIN
AND DNA IN L-1210 CELLS:*
    It seems that the biological basis of malignant growth
lies in the active biosynthesis of protein and nucleic acids.
Therefore, the effect of harringtonine on the biosynthesis of
protein and DNA in L-1210 cells was studied.
    By means of autoradiography, the incorporation efficien-
cies of ^{3}H-L-Asparagin into tumor cells of the control group
were compared with those of the treated group. Experimental
results showed that one intraperitoneal injection of 1 mg/kg
of harringtonine caused a significant inhibition of protein
synthesis. The incorporation of ^{3}H-TdR into DNA was also
affected profoundly.

6. *CYTOKINETIC EFFECT OF HARRINGTONINE ON L-1210 CELLS:*
    There is an increasing body of knowledge on the cyto-
kinetic effect of anticancer agents. Such studies may prove
to be an important therapeutic lead to clinical trials.
Therefore we investigated the cytokinetic effect of harringtonine on L-1210 cells.
    (1) Autoradiographic Studies
        1) *Pulse-labeling Experiments*
    Thirty minutes after a single intraperitoneal injection
of 20μci of ^{3}H-TdR into L-1210 bearing mice, harringtonine
was injected intraperitoneally into each mouse. Five hours
later, the ascitic cells were collected, smeared and stained
by Giemsa stain. Experiments revealed that under the action
of harringtonine a number of nuclei of L-1210 cells had dis-
integrated into several fragments. The percentage of
labeled damaged cells reached 26.1%, whereas the nonlabeled
damaged one was only 11.9% by the fifth hour after the treatment. At the moment, the labeled index was lowered significantly. These results meant that the tumor cells in the S
phase were seriously damaged.
        2) *Continuous Labeling Experiments:*
    ^{3}H-TdR was injected every two hours for 16 hours into
L-1210 bearing mice. Experiments demonstrated that on the
seventh day after the implantation of L-1210 cells into DBA/2
mice the 60 cells amounted to 52% of the cell population.
Under the action of harringtonine, nearly 37% of the Go cells
had sustained serious morphological damage.
    (2) Colchicine Amide Blockade Experiments:
    Experiments showed that under the action of colchicine

amide, the mitotic index of L-1210 cells increased sharply.
However the combination of harringtonine and colchicine amide
caused only a slight increase of mitotic index in L-1210
cells. This fact indicates that under the action of harringtonine, the progression of the cell in G_2 phase into M phase
was blocked.

    (3) <u>Cytophotometric Measurement of DNA Content per Cell</u>:
It is well known that the DNA content per cell distribu-
tions yield direct information regarding the frequency of
cells outside the S compartment. Therefore, the fractions of
cells in G_1, S, and G_2 plus M phases can be determined from
the DNA histogram of these cells. With the aid of an MPV II
microscopic photometer, the DNA content per cell of a control
group and a treated group were compared. At a dosage of
20µg per mouse, harringtonine induced a significant decrease
of L-1210 cells in S phase, while cells in G_1 phase were
increased and a new peak appeared in the low channel. This
means that under the action of the drug, the traverse of the
leukemic cells in G_1 phase into S phase was blocked.

    (4) <u>Cinemicrographic Studies</u>:
Murine leukemia L-1210 and P-388 cells and a line of
human acute myelocytic leukemia cells (J6-1) were cultivated
aseptically in the medium of RPMI-1640, with 10% calf-serum
added. By means of the Nikon inverted microscope Model MD,
equipped with incubator and cine camera, the dynamic morphological changes of L-1210 and P-388 cells treated with
harringtonine were photographed every 8 seconds on a negative
16 mm film. Before the addition of harringtonine, the leukemic cells were intact morphologically, and their movement
was less active. Under high magnification, the movement of
the nuclei and mitochondria of the cells was visible.

    At a concentration of 30µg/ml for 30 minutes, harring-
tonine initially accelerated the movement of L-1210 cells
and succeeded in a disruption of cell membrane and resulted
in karyorrhexis. After 3 hours, a large number of leukemic
cells died and the movement of these cells stopped. But the
cells in mitosis remained intact and could complete their
mitotic process. The morphological changes in human leukemic
cells were essentially the same as in murine leukemic cells.

7. *PHYSIOLOGICAL DISPOSITION OF HARRINGTONINE*:
    Absorption, distribution and excretion patterns were
studied on rats. After an intravenous injection of [3]H-
harringtonine (200µci/kg), various biological specimens were
collected and their radioactivities counted by a liquid
scintillation counter.

    Experiments disclosed that 15 minutes after intravenous
injection, the labeled drug was distributed mainly in the

following organs: kidney, liver, bone marrow, lung, heart, gastrointestinal tract, spleen and salivary glands.

Two hours later, the radioactivity in these organs decreased significantly, except for the bone marrow, which remained at a higher level. The half-life ($t\frac{1}{2}$) of the radioactivity in the plasma of rats can be divided into two phases: fast phase (3.5 minutes) and slow phase (50 minutes). The total excretion of radioactivity from urine in the first 24 hours amounted to 30.2% of the administered dose, of which about 12.9% was unchanged drug. The remainder was its metabolite. The excretion from feces in the first 24 hours amounted to 16.6%, of which 1.6% was found to be unchanged. The macro-autoradiographic studies showed similar results.

8. *INFLUENCE OF HARRINGTONINE ON IMMUNE RESPONSES:*

In view of the fact that the majority of antineoplastic agents were immunosuppressants, we studied the effect of harringtonine on the immunological competence of mice. By using the hemolytic plaque-forming cell assays developed by Jerne et al., and the graft versus host reaction, the influence of the drug on the immune responses was investigated. Experiments demonstrated that at the therapeutic dosage harringtonine decreased the number of hemolytic plaque-forming cells and reduced the spleen index of the hosts.

9. *COMPARISON OF THE FOUR ESTERS OF CEPHALOTAXINE:*

By means of conventional microscopy and autoradiography, the cytokinetic effects of partial synthetic harringtonine, homoharringtonine, isoharringtonine and deoxyharringtonine were compared at the comparable dosage in L-1210 bearing mice. Cytological examination demonstrated that partial synthetic harringtonine and homoharringtonine decreased the mitotic index of L-1210 cells significantly and the deoxy-harringtonine exhibited lesser effect, while isoharringtonine did not affect the MI of the leukemic cells. The effect of the four esters on the incorporation of radiolabeled precursors into the nuclei of L-1210 cells was compared by autoradiography. In comparing the action of these four esters of cephalotaxine, we found that the incorporation of ^{3}H-TdR into nuclei of L-1210 cells was inhibited most markedly by homoharringtonine, followed by harringtonine, deoxyharringtonine and isoharringtonine. As for the effect on the cells in S phase experiments showed that the partial synthetic harringtonine and homoharringtonine decreased the LI more effectively than other esters of cephalotaxine. These results illustrate that partial synthetic harringtonine and homoharringtonine are more efficient esters of cephalotaxine than others.

B. CLINICAL STUDIES

In 1974, on the basis of preclinical toxicological
studies, harringtonine was introduced to phase 1 study. In
phase 2 study, the drug was used as a single agent, at a
dosage of 0.2 mg/kg for seven consecutive days, followed by
a 7-15 day rest. In the course of treatment, harringtonine
was dissolved in 500 ml of 10% glucose solution and administered by slow intravenous drip. The most promising results
were observed in cases of acute myelocytic leukemia.
Thirteen cases (28%) out of 47 achieved complete remission
and 27 cases (57%) achieved partial remission. The total
remission rate was about 85%. The response of acute monocytic leukemia to this drug was also encouraging. A complete
remission which lasted more than two years, was noted in one
case of erythroleukemia. It was also discussed to be effective in acute lymphocytic leukemia and blast crisis of
chronic myelocytic leukemia.

DISCUSSION AND SUMMARY

Apparently, the genetic relationship of plants were
formed during the evolutionary process. Therefore, closely
related species, which belong to the same genus, may contain
similar chemical components. This may serve as a lead in
the search for new drugs.
There are eight species of the Cephalotaxus plant in
China, among which Cephalotaxus fortunei Hook F is the most
abundant and widely distributed. Cephalotaxus sinensis Li
and Cephalotaxus oliveri Mast are also common and plentiful.
Cephalotaxus hainanensis Li is indigenous to Hainan Island,
in the Kwangtung province. In the latter plant, the content
of the esters of cephalotaxine is the highest among related
species.
In recent years, we have studied Cephalotaxus hainanensis Li, from which several active antitumor principles were
isolated and characterized. Pharmacological studies demonstrated that harringtonine is an inhibitor of protein and DNA
synthesis. It is a cell cycle nonspecific agent in cytokinetic effects. Ultrastructural studies showed that harringtonine induced a peculiar karyorrhexis in L-1210 cells.
After intravenous injection, harringtonine was distributed
mainly in the kidney, liver, lungs, G.I. tract, spleen, bone
marrow and salivary glands. On the basis of preclinical
toxicological studies, harringtonine was introduced into
clinical trials, which yielded promising results in the
treatment of acute myelocytic leukemia, acute monocytic

leukemia, and erythroleukemia. Now, harringtonine is being used widely in clinics in China, and over 300 patients suffering from leukemias or lymphomas have been treated with this drug.

Because of the plant's meager content of harringtonine and the increasing clinical demand for it, the study of its partial synthesis was carried out by chemists in our Institute. With levulinic acid as the starting material through seven steps of reactions, they succeeded in preparing the desired compound, a mixture of two diastereoisomers, harringtonine and epiharringtonine, separable with partition column chromatography. Experimental chemotherapeutic studies revealed that the partial synthetic harringtonine was as active in rodent tumors as natural harringtonine. Toxicological studies showed that the LD_{50} of the synthetic mixture was twice that of the natural harringtonine. These results coincided well with the chemical features. On the basis of preclinical toxicological studies, the partial synthetic diastereoisomers have entered into clinical trial, and further works are in progress.

The study of Cephalotaxus hainanensis Li illustrates our approach to obtain new antitumor agents from plants. Cancer is a worldwide enemy of mankind. Although substantial advances have been made in the treatment of malignant diseases, the conquest of cancer remains a great challenge. We are sure that close, international cooperation among scientific communities will greatly accelerate the development of anticancer agents.

Index

269

272

a
b
c
d
e
f
g
h
1 i
8 2 j